Slim

THE ITALIAN WAY

A Weight-Loss Surgeon's
Guide to Losing Weight

Eldo E. Frezza MD, MBA, FACS

Slim

THE ITALIAN WAY

is published by
Ciné-Med, Inc.

ISBN: 978-0-9749358-8-1

Cover Art
Ed Freeman
Cara Forbes

Printed in Canada
2nd Edition

Dedication

This book is dedicated to my children, Edoardo and Gianmarco
and my wife Patrizia, who helped with the recipe section of this book
and fills our family kitchen with love and great food.

A particular dedication goes to my mother, Rosa,
for the many suggestions on diet while I grew up in Italy, which
are reported in this book, and to my father, Giovanni.

A special thanks goes to my editor, June Grace Wagner
whose guidance has been invaluable.

Contents

Introduction

The Italian Philosophy of Diet

The Science of Food

Ladies and Gentlemen, Start your Diet!

Recipes   "From our family to you"

Meat & Poultry

Desserts

Appendices

Eating Should Be Pleasant, Not Inflict Guilt or Self-Loathing

Food can and should give us happiness and pleasure.

Every day in my practice as a surgeon specializing in treating the overweight, I encounter patients whose weight problems have literally put their lives in danger. These are men and women who are so morbidly obese that surgery is often the only solution. They are also individuals who have tried every kind of diet and are filled with guilt and self-loathing. And why? When you look at the available diet and weight loss books, the majority of them blame the reader for eating too much or for indulging in the wrong foods. And while most of these books tell you what to avoid eating, they do not tell you what to eat or how to eat. Nor do they provide sound, healthful principles for losing weight.

As a consequence, dieters come to view food with fear, as a temptation that must be conquered through deprivation and mind-numbing self-control. Those who cannot control their hunger are left with a feeling of failure and a conviction that they are incapable of managing their own lives.

We Are Losing the Battle

While few of us will ever need surgery to achieve a healthy weight, it is no secret that we are losing the battle to control our weight. Why? One of the problems with diets is that most of them are too strict, limiting not only the quantity of intake, but the quality as well. In their zeal to promote new ways to lose weight, they rob us of one of life's most basic enjoyments.

I believe that food is something that can and should give us happiness and pleasure. Part of this belief stems from my upbringing in Italy, where people are much less conflicted about food. If you go to Italy, people seem very happy, and this happiness is in large part related to what they eat.

What Are We Going to Cook Today?

Whenever I visit my family in Venice, one of the main questions is, "What are we going to cook today?" This question is asked at 7:30 in the morning, while we are eating breakfast and drinking coffee. It may seem strange that decisions about lunch or dinner are made at this

A National Epidemic

Obesity has become a national epidemic. Not only are a majority of adult Americans overweight, some 50 percent of us, but so are an increasing number of our children. The proportion of overweight children has tripled since 1980. These startling numbers mean that we are at increased risk for a whole host of health problems associated with excess weight: diabetes, high blood pressure, and heart disease, to name just a few.

hour of the morning, but this reflects our respect for food and its preparation. In Italy, it is never too early to start planning a meal!

Dinner should be seen as a happy conclusion to the day, not as an event to be dreaded. There are few things that make people happier than family, friends, food, and the rituals which celebrate such fellowship in the presence of good food. The Italian diet is characterized by fresh, colorful, and varied ingredients, and good taste. There is an innate joy and spirit of adventure in having different types of meals to cook every day, an undertaking easily accomplished since the ingredients of Italian cooking are extremely basic.

The goals are to maintain

• a healthy body

• a healthy weight

and to

• repossess the adventure and joy of eating.

Food, A Key to Happiness

The Italians and the peoples of the Mediterranean use food as a key to happiness and, if used correctly, it can also be the key to losing weight. My experience as a surgeon has convinced me that we need to find a way to lose weight while preserving one of the great pleasures of life, and that is what this book is all about. We need to continue to enjoy the pleasure of eating while teaching our body to understand when and how we need to eat and what foods we need to eat.

Food Is Not Evil

Let's go back to the basics of food intake. Food is not evil, it is a pleasure. As the Romans once said, food is a gift from the gods. This book will give you the tools to lose weight safely and effectively while still eating happily.

How are we going to achieve that?

• First, we will suggest an eating schedule that respects the needs of your body. To accomplish this, we will need to understand some of the basics of digestion—

  - why food works in certain ways,
  - why we get so hungry,
  - why we feel that we need more food and
  - what we can do to eliminate those feelings.

• Second, we will provide some light, flavorful recipes that are easy to prepare and will supply you with both nutrition and sensory enjoyment.

From: Susan, New Mexico

I went to see Dr. Frezza regarding undergoing bariatric surgery, but I was not 100 pounds overweight so my insurance would not cover the surgery. I then asked Dr. Frezza to design a diet for me. He gave me his own diet and after two weeks, I saw major results. I was able to understand my problem, which became clear to me after reading his diet philosophy. I was able to apply the principles he suggested and lost 23 pounds in the first month. I believe the most important thing that I learned from his diet is the importance of taking care of ourselves and making food our friend. We can enjoy eating and not gain weight.

Honesty: The First Step Toward Losing Weight

The first step to losing weight is being completely honest about how far off you are from a healthy weight.

Patients who come to me for obesity surgery often confide in me things they would not tell their families or friends. They are frank and come straight to the point: they do not want to die of a heart attack or a stroke like their mother or their grandfather.

What invariably moves me about my patients is how they have come to grips with the fact that they are overweight and know that they must change if they are going to achieve a better quality of life. They tell me they want to be able to play with their children or grandchildren and see them reach adulthood. Or they tell me they want to get married again, find a better job, or travel to a place they've always dreamed of—Italy or maybe Madagascar. Regardless of their motivation, they all share one common trait: they have faced their problem and made a conscious choice to improve their lives.

Obesity Is Preventable

The good news about obesity is that it is preventable. In fact, obesity and overweight are considered the number one most preventable cause of death in the United States. Thirty-one percent, or approximately 59 million Americans over the age of 20, are obese.

Looking in a mirror or standing on a scale may give you a rough understanding of how many pounds you need to lose. If you are a woman, you may notice that fat has tended to collect around the buttocks and thighs and given you a pear-shaped appearance. If you are a man, you will notice that fat has collected mostly around the belly and given you an apple-shaped appearance. However, let's get more precise about your weight. The best way to determine how overweight you are is to measure your weight in relation to your height. This measurement, known as the body mass index, BMI, is the measurement of choice for most physicians and researchers studying obesity. BMI uses a mathematical formula that takes into account both a person's height and weight.

Definition

Overweight	10 to 30	pounds over a healthy weight.
Obese	30 to 100	pounds over a healthy weight.
Morbidly obese	100+	pounds over a healthy body weight.

Calculate Your BMI

Please use the following table to determine how overweight you are. It's simple! The table has already calculated all the math and metric conversions. All you have to do is find your height in inches in the left-hand column, then move across the row to the your weight in pounds. The number at the top of that column is the BMI for that height and weight.

Determining Your Body Mass Index (BMI)

BMI (kg/m2)	19	20	21	22	23	24	25	26	27	28	29	30	35	40
Height in inches	Weight in pounds													
58	91	96	100	105	110	115	119	124	129	134	138	143	167	191
59	94	99	104	109	114	119	124	128	133	138	143	148	173	198
60	97	102	107	112	118	123	128	133	138	143	148	153	179	204
61	100	106	111	116	122	127	132	137	143	148	153	158	185	211
62	104	109	115	120	126	131	136	142	147	153	158	164	191	218
63	107	113	118	124	130	135	141	146	152	158	163	169	197	225
64	110	116	122	128	134	140	145	151	157	163	169	174	204	232
65	114	120	126	132	138	144	150	156	162	168	174	180	210	240
66	118	124	130	136	142	148	155	161	167	173	179	186	216	247
67	121	127	134	140	146	153	159	166	172	178	185	191	223	255
68	125	131	138	144	151	158	164	171	177	184	190	197	230	262
69	128	135	142	149	155	162	169	176	182	189	196	203	236	270
70	132	139	146	153	160	167	174	181	188	195	202	207	243	278
71	136	143	150	157	165	172	179	186	193	200	208	215	250	286
72	140	147	154	162	169	177	184	191	199	206	213	221	258	294
73	144	151	159	166	174	182	189	197	204	212	219	227	265	302
74	148	155	163	171	179	186	194	202	210	218	225	233	272	311
75	152	160	168	176	184	192	200	208	216	224	232	240	279	319
76	156	164	172	180	189	197	205	213	221	230	238	246	287	328

Body weight in pounds according to height and body mass index.
Adapted from Bray, G.A., Gray, D.S.,Obesity, Part I,
Pathogenesis, West J. Med. 1988: 149: 429-41.

At your ideal weight, you'll have more energy and enthusiasm for both current and new activities. And isn't that what life is all about?

If you did not find your BMI, it means your BMI is above 40. You might want to refer to the Internet using, for example, the BMI Calculator of obesityhelp.com.

Now that you have calculated your BMI, let's see what the number actually means. The National Institute of Health considers individuals between 20 and 25 BMI to be of normal weight, those between 25 and 30 BMI to be overweight, those between 30 and 35 BMI to be obese, those between 35 and 40 BMI to be moderately obese, and those with a BMI over 40 to be morbidly obese.

For example, a 5 foot 6 inch person who weighs 161 pounds would be overweight, while a person of the same height who weighs 186 pounds is obese.

How Much Weight Do You Need to Lose?

To find how much weight you need to lose, find the weight for a BMI of 25 for your height.

If your weight is that weight or less, congratulations! You do not need to lose any pounds! This diet program will help you maintain an optimum weight and a healthy body, too.

If your weight is greater than the BMI 25 weight for your height, subtract that weight from your actual weight. The answer is how many pounds you need to lose.

Now let us begin to learn how to change your eating patterns. It is important to remember that losing weight is not going to make your life perfect. However, it will improve your quality of life and enable you to look and feel better.

Body Mass Index (BMI) Summary

Normal	BMI of 20-25
Overweight	BMI of 25-30
Obese	BMI of 30-35
Moderately Obese	BMI of 35-40
Morbidly Obese	BMI of 40+

"Viva la vita!"
as the Italians say.
In English, this means
"Cheers to a good life!"

Real Expectations Will Yield Real Results

Many people plunge into a weight loss program with great enthusiasm and are able to lose 20, 30, even 50 pounds. But what happens in the months afterwards?

People's expectations fall into one of three categories:

1) They are going to maintain the weight loss;

2) They are going to gain some weight back; or

3) They do not care what is going to happen after they lose the weight, they just want to lose it now!

Dieters often lose sight of the unfortunate fact that most of the time when they diet, they regain the weight, and, often, gain even more. Why does this happen?

Weight Loss Is Stressful

The body sees weight loss as a stressor and will try to gain more weight to defend itself against another stressful situation, thus preventing it from losing weight. Keep in mind that throughout most of human history, food has been scarce rather than plentiful. Our bodies have adapted to perceive any reduction in food intake as a signal of famine. Thus, when food is readily available, we will load up on calories in preparation for the next shortage. While all this helped ensure the survival of human beings over the centuries, it is not very helpful in our modern society of abundance.

Since your body has been adapted to your particular lifestyle for a long time, it will perceive any weight loss as a disruption to its equilibrium. Whenever it has the chance to gain weight, it will try to regain it.

It is important, therefore, to specify and set your goals before attempting to lose weight. Do you want to lose 5, 10, or 20 pounds?

Having a goal in mind, working to reach that goal, and maintaining that goal are very important. Setting a goal of how much you want to lose, however, is not as important as keeping the weight off because, as we've seen, that is the most difficult thing to do. You need to have a plan of action for keeping the weight loss permanent. You should not starve yourself to death for three months to lose 20 pounds and then start eating as much as you can for the next three months because you will gain all of the weight right back.

Write down your goal and post it in a prominent place…the refrigerator, the bathroom mirror, or your daily calendar.

We should also carefully evaluate the food we eat and give our families. We need to change our eating patterns and choose healthier foods. By smarter choices, we can teach our children, husbands, and wives to eat healthy types of food. These foods will then be what we find on our tables and in our refrigerators.

One of the easiest ways to reach this goal is simply to shop smarter.

The Key to permanent weight loss is a permanent change in eating patterns and food choices

Shop the Perimeter

If you look at the set-up of most supermarkets in the United States, you will notice that they share a common attribute: to find the healthy, low-calorie foods, you must stay on the perimeter of the supermarket, where the vegetables, fruit, meat, and milk products are located. If you walk through the middle aisles, you will find baked goods, sodas, sweets, and other highly processed foods. Therefore, train yourself to shop mostly along the perimeter of the supermarket.

Why Do We Overeat?

1) Stress

Before undertaking a diet program, we also need to try to understand some of the psychological reasons we tend to overeat. Loss of a relative, going through a divorce, or other personal or professional problems are often reasons for gaining weight, but they cannot become a permanent reason for overeating. Like many people, I tend to eat more during a stressful situation. For example, I gained weight while studying for my medical exam when my usual eating patterns were disrupted by late-night studying and snacking. After the exam was over, however, my life went back to normal and I returned to my original weight.

Stress

If you are currently enduring a major stressful situation, you need to resolve it before making any other changes in your life. Make goals about what to do when the stressful situation is relieved.

2) Bad Habits

A lot of overeating, however, simply stems from falling into bad habits, such as eating too many high-calorie foods or snacking in front of the television. In these cases, taking note of what we eat and how much, can be truly eye-opening.

3) Behavioral

The quantity of food we tend to eat is largely a behavioral response to our surroundings and to what other people do. This is why obesity tends to be common in families who share similar food choices and eating habits. It is well known that the problem of morbid obesity is a behavioral and social problem. In general, fried foods will make us hungrier; therefore, we tend to keep eating these foods.

Morbid obesity is a behavioral and social problem.

Be Aware of the Foods You Eat

It is important, therefore, to be aware of the foods you are consuming. Get a notebook or use the form in Chapter 16 and write down the food you eat; you will be surprised! When you undertake a diet, you want to focus on making healthier food choices that will enable you to lose weight simply and gradually. In this way, you will best be able to achieve success.

Women with Children

Many women who have children say that one of the reasons they gain weight is because they clean their children's plates. Whatever the kids do not eat, they eat because they cannot bear to throw the food away. Thus, they end up eating a lot of macaroni and cheese and French fries. My response to this is, "Why feed your children foods high in carbohydrates and sugar when that will only make them obese teenagers?"

The Point:
Do not give your children foods
you do not want to eat yourself.

Understanding How Your Stomach Works

Focus on making healthier food choices.

In the 1980s, the Royal British Army had a major problem. The soldiers kept complaining about their meals, saying that they did not like the food and that they never felt full. The British evaluated several alternatives and came up with a Mediterranean style diet for the troops. Initially, there was much joking. Why, people asked, were the queen's soldiers being fed Italian food?

The explanation is very simple and interesting. The soldiers needed food that tasted good but, at the same time, they needed food that would fill them up until their next meal. The choice of an Italian diet was based on the fact that not only is Italian food flavorful, but it is filling because there is a sufficient quantity of proteins and carbohydrates to prevent our stomachs from requiring more food. Let's evaluate why this is so important to our weight loss program.

Digestion

It is important to recognize that eating is only one part of our daily routine; the process of digestion continues well after we have physically left the table. Because the stomach is a strong muscle, it physically churns food to shreds and then liquefies it with the aid of potent gastric juices and acid. After the food has been broken down in the stomach, it passes into the small intestine, where it is absorbed into the bloodstream, largely as carbohydrates, fat and proteins.

The Amazing Stomach

The stomach plays a key role in our ability to lose weight, but few people really understand how this amazing organ works and its role in feelings of hunger or fullness. First of all, it is important to understand that the stomach is a muscle; therefore, it has a tendency to expand or adjust to its full capacity. In many years of performing surgery, I have found that the stomachs of obese patients tend to be larger than those of the non-obese. The stomach is able to adapt itself to new situations and tries to accommodate an individual by growing. These actual anatomical changes occur gradually over several years as a result of the amount of food eaten.

There are ways to slow down the digestive process and decrease feelings of hunger. Eating something raw, like cauliflower or broccoli, increases the amount of time it takes for the stomach to digest it. Cooking, on the other hand, helps break down food and speeds the digestive process. The more highly processed and sugar laden a food is, the faster the stomach digests it and passes it into the bloodstream. The faster the food enters the bloodstream, the more quickly you will become hungry again. To understand how this works, you need to know something about how insulin regulates blood sugar.

Insulin

Insulin is the main hormone that controls how much sugar there is in the bloodstream. In healthy people, whenever there is increased sugar in the bloodstream, the pancreas produces insulin, which lowers the amount of sugar in the blood by getting the cells of various organs to absorb sugar.

In a disease called type 1 diabetes, the pancreas does not secrete any insulin. Patients who develop this disease might die without intake of artificial insulin because the amount of sugar in the blood quickly rises to intolerable levels.

In type 2 diabetes, on the other hand, the cells do not respond as well as they should to insulin's orders to absorb blood sugar, meaning that the body must secrete more insulin to achieve the same result. The medical term for this is "insulin resistance." In most obese patients, some degree of insulin resistance is always present. One reason that obesity surgery works is that it reduces insulin resistance.

In healthy people the pancreas is able to produce the appropriate amounts of insulin. The faster the digestive process sends sugar into the bloodstream, the more quickly the pancreas responds to produce insulin. The faster the insulin goes into the bloodstream, the more quickly the sugar level decreases. Decreases in blood sugar tell the body it is time to eat again. This is why you feel hungrier if you eat foods that the stomach can quickly digest. To decrease the hunger urge, we need to eat food that the stomach will take time to process.

If you eat foods that make you feel full for longer periods of time, you will be able to lose weight without feelings of hunger.

To decrease hunger, eat foods that take time to digest i.e.foods that are raw or have lots of fiber like raw vegetables and fruit.

In his book, *The South Beach Diet*, Dr. Agatston uses the example of a baked potato. Baking the potato enables it to enter the digestive system more quickly. However, if we put sour cream on the potato, this will slow down the digestive process. The same concept applies to a toasted bagel in the morning. The process of toasting will help the food to be digested. But if you add some cream cheese, this will slow down the digestion of the bagel. If there is nothing to slow down the process of digestion, we will want food an hour or two after we have eaten.

Fiber

Fiber is an excellent way to slow down the digestive process because it takes time for the stomach to break down the fiber. For example, if you eat a pear without fiber, such as a canned pear, versus a pear with fiber, such as an unpeeled, fresh pear, digestion can vary from a half hour to more than an hour, respectively. Therefore, you are going to feel hungry again after an hour versus two hours. If you eat foods that make you feel full for longer periods of time, you will be able to lose weight without feelings of hunger.

Achieving well–being and a healthy body weight involves the proper balance of carbohydrates, fats, and proteins, a balance which is inherent in the Italian diet.

An Italian Discovering Italian Food in America

The Mediterranean diet was probably the first diet ever used to lose weight. In the long history of European conquests, many foreign conquerors came to Italy, appreciated the local food, and frequently imported the cuisine back to their own countries. Yet when I first came to America, I was surprised by how differently Italian cuisine is perceived and prepared in the U.S. In the U.S., Italian cuisine is viewed as a high-fat, high-calorie indulgence with rich sauces and cheeses, which is not a perfect mirror of Italian food in Italy.

When Americans think of Italian cuisine, however, they think primarily of pizza and pasta. But if you order a pepperoni pizza in Italy, you are going to be served a pizza with peppers because "peperoni" is the Italian word for peppers. Pepperoni pizza did not originate in Italy. This fatty combination came from Brooklyn and has spread throughout the United States as an "Italian" specialty.

What strikes you most when you go to Italy is how much smaller the portions are.

Super-Sizing

The problems with Americanized Italian cuisine stem from modifying the original recipes and then super-sizing them. In America, we are used to having super-sized portions. We simply don't realize how much bigger the portion sizes are in comparison to those served throughout Europe. In Italy, a typical serving of pasta is about 60 grams, just short of 2 ounces. It does not cover an entire plate; it barely fills the bottom half of a normal-sized pasta plate.

Adapt Your Stomach

The most important thing is to adapt your stomach to eating less. In fact, the key to my diet is to decrease the amount of food you eat at mealtimes and eat the foods you enjoy in moderation, so that you will not distend your stomach further than you should. The Italian diet will help you to enjoy a variety of foods that taste good without limiting you to just a few food choices during the day. The goal is to lose weight at a steady pace because this is best for your health, as well as best for acquiring new eating habits. If you need to lose weight more quickly, I have provided a four-phase diet in Appendix 3 that I give to my patients after they have had surgery. Please remember that this is a much more drastic diet that was designed to help my patients adjust from having a big stomach to a small stomach. It may not suit people with limited weight-loss needs.

When you eat less, the stomach gets used to receiving less food, and when you receive more food than you are accustomed, you will experience discomfort. This discomfort will help you in the diet process because when you feel it, you will understand that your stomach is not used to eating that amount of food any more; therefore, you will stop eating such large amounts. In this way, you can moderate your intake of food without cheating and without decreasing the pleasure of eating.

Fresh Ingredients

What most Americans may not realize is the emphasis the traditional Italian diet places on fresh fruit and vegetables. One of the most wonderful things about Italy is the large open-air markets, where people come from the countryside, particularly farmers, to sell their fruits and vegetables. When I was growing up in Venice, people were proud of eating fresh fruit every day. It was a pleasure during lunchtime, when offices were closed and school was out, to stop and buy fresh fruit and vegetables or to stop by the dairy shop for some fresh mozzarella or ricotta. The portion sizes were just enough for lunch or dinner, but never enough for two or three days because we, like most Italians, did not have a large refrigerator.

Fresh fish is another traditional staple of the Italian diet. Hence, fresh fish markets are another common sight in Italy. The one in Venice dates back to the time when the city first became an independent republic. Set in an open space with multiple columns, the market is a magnificent place to view the fish the fisherman have caught during the night and brought to sell that morning. You can find every type of fish from the Adriatic Sea displayed on the large tables.

My aunt, who lives in Naples, loves to visit the fish market in her city. One time when I was visiting her, we bought some fresh octopus. When we returned to her home, we cleaned it, boiled it, and then sliced it into a tomato sauce with a little onion and garlic. The result? A simple, low-fat dish packed with gourmet flavor. One thing Italians know is that the fresher your ingredients are, the more flavorful your meal will be and the less need you will have to smother your dish with caloric sauces.

> The goal in learning new eating patterns is to teach your stomach to enjoy food in a normal, healthy capacity, without overstuffing it.

Added Calories and Fat

One of the problems with the Italian cuisine in America is that more butter, cheese, or sauce is added to make the food "taste better." As a result, many Italian-American recipes are richer than the original version. For example, in Italy pasta is delicately coated with sauce, while in the U.S., the ratio is inverted, and too often pasta is served swimming in large amounts of sauce.

Italian-American restaurants also love to perpetuate the myth that Italians end every meal with a rich and decadent dessert. While it may be true that one of the Italy's greatest gifts to the world are its sweets such as tiramisú, gelato and cannoli, to name a few, Italians prefer to end meals on a very light note. A small bowl of fresh fruit or a tablespoon or two of homemade sorbet is the most that even the most enterprising Italian cook will present at the end of a meal.

The rich and large-portioned desserts with which Italian-American restaurants tempt their customers are, instead, treats that Italians prefer to reserve for special occasions such as a holiday meal, a birthday, or a weekend treat.

The Problems with Italian Cuisine in the U.S.

1. The portions are larger or super-sized.
2. Fresh ingredients like fruits and vegetables have been reduced or eliminated from dishes; or when they are served, they come with a high-sugar content dipping cream.
3. Modifications from the original recipes have led to completely different recipes that are higher in calories.

The Italian Philosophy

The Italians may live their lives around their tables, but they are thinner because of their food choices and their portion sizes.

Coming together at the table is something done in Italy by simply putting food on the table and eating. It is a sensory and social experience, a way to share thoughts and emotions. Every time families get together in Italy, food is the primary way of entertaining. It is essential to our social fabric, our way of life. Fresh fruits, vegetables, and fish, as well as pasta and olive oil, are the basic components of the traditional Italian diet. Not only do they keep our weight in check, but they also confer enormous health benefits.

Contrary to popular belief, most Italians are not overweight. If you travel to Italy or the surrounding Mediterranean region, you will see that most of the young men and women are slim and trim. Their parents and grandparents also look healthy and fit. You can see certain ranges of obesity, but nowhere do you see the extremes of obesity so common in the United States.

What is the secret of the Italians? They follow a very simple rule: they eat a balanced diet in small portions. A balanced diet will not only help you to control your desire to overeat, but it will also allow you to eat the correct amount of proteins, carbohydrates, and vitamins that are necessary for health in your daily life.

Balance

The Italian diet is not only a low-fat diet, but it is a diet that teaches you how to regulate your intake of carbohydrates, fats, and proteins. It enables you to live happily with your choices and not to worry about the food you eat after the meal. You can eat a normal-sized portion of meat or fish, including beef, chicken, pork, turkey, fish, lamb, or shellfish. You can eat preferentially all of the green vegetables and tomatoes, excluding other colored vegetables. You can eat cheese, eggs, and nuts. By following the Italian diet, you will regain the pleasure of sitting at the table. There is no extreme deprivation involved in this diet; you will be able to enjoy three balanced meals with a snack in between meals.

The benefits of the Italian and Mediterranean diets are supported by decades of research. An early pioneer on the effect of diet and lifestyle on health was the physiologist, Ancel Keys. In the 1950s, he conducted his now famous "Seven Countries Study," which compared the diets of people between the ages of 40 and 60 from such diverse parts of the world as Japan, the U.S., Italy, former

Yugoslavia, Finland, the Netherlands, and Greece.

Keys found that poor heart health was more prevalent in countries where the amounts of fats, carbohydrates, and proteins were consumed in excessive amounts, as they are in the U.S. On the other hand, in countries where olive oil, cereals, vegetables, fruits, and fish made up the bulk of the foods consumed, the risk of heart attacks and coronary disease was greatly reduced. This was a revolutionary discovery because at that time scientists believed the levels of fat in the body were fixed and unchangeable, rather than dependent on diet.

In general, your meals should consist of 55–60% carbohydrates, 20% protein, and 25–30% fat.

Over the years, arteriosclerosis, hypertension, heart attack, stroke, and diabetes have all been shown to decrease with a Mediterranean diet. A study performed by the Disability Adjusted Life Expectancy (DALE) Agency analyzed longevity in many different countries. The U.S. ranked 24th and Italy ranked 5th. A French study performed in Saint Etienne found that only 14 patients who were following the Mediterranean diet died in four years. In contrast, 24 patients who did not follow the Mediterranean diet died. In the Mediterranean diet group, there were 50% less cancers and 33% less heart attacks than in groups following other types of diets.

What accounted for the drastic differences in death rates? The omega-3 fatty acids found in fish oil and olive oil, both of which are major components in the Mediterranean diet, accounted in large part for the extended longevity of the participants in the study.

A Healthy Lifestyle

The Italian diet emphasizes making healthy food choices rather than counting calories, which is not always easy to do. For example, if I follow a recipe, and I use Cheese A instead of Cheese B, does Cheese A have the same number of calories as Cheese B? I have bought foods at different supermarkets and realized that the caloric content of the basic ingredients is different. The Italian diet allows us to avoid this issue and focus on more general food groups.

The daily beverage recommendation is a minimum of eight glasses of water, preferably one gallon, or any other fluid without sugar, and wine in moderation.

Research has shown that a lot of fruit and vegetables eaten every day, together with bread, pasta, or rice are important. You also need to avoid excessive amounts of alcohol and engage in moderate physical activity (at least 30 minutes per day). All these things contribute to a lifestyle that has been shown to reduce cancer as well as heart disease and diabetes.

Diet and Cancer

Because of the strong link that has been found between cancer and lifestyle, some physicians consider cancer to be an environmental disease. "Environmental" includes everything in our surroundings, such as the air we breathe, the water we drink, and the food we eat.

Food is the fundamental, controllable component in our lives. We can choose what we eat, but we cannot choose what we breathe. There are many antioxidants in vegetables and fruits that are able to block certain deadly chemical reactions. Research has shown that vegetables and fruits help fight carcinogenic agents. For instance, in the mouth, larynx, esophagus, stomach, and intestines, some tumors are the result of a chemical reaction to certain foods, alcohol, and tobacco. It has been shown that there is a direct relation between increased cancer risk and a diet lacking in fruit and vegetables. At the same time, there is a direct correlation between a diet of saturated fat (fat from animals) and some forms of cancer, such as gastrointestinal and breast cancers.

The Basics of the Italian Philosophy

Daily physical activity.

Daily intake of 8 or more glasses of water.

Daily intake of bread, pasta, rice or other whole grains, and/or a potato.

Daily intake of vegetables.

Daily intake of fresh fruits.

Daily intake of olive oil.

Daily intake of cheese.

Moderate alcohol consumption.

Weekly intake of fish.

Weekly intake of poultry.

Weekly intake of eggs.

Weekly intake of sweets.

Bi-monthly intake of red meat.

Based on these findings, the European Society for the Research of Cancer recommends the daily food intake to include:

1. Two portions of pasta or rice, with minimal sauce;

2. Two portions of vegetables, either cooked or fresh;

3. Two or three servings of fruit per day;

4. Two glasses of milk or yogurt; and

5. Boiled fish, meat, beans, cheese, or an egg.

As you can see, their list coincides with the findings of the Mediterranean diet.

Water, Before and After Each Meal

Also central to the modified Italian diet is water. You will need to drink at least one gallon of water per day including your favorite drinks. One suggestion I learned from my mother is to drink one or two cups of water or other low-calorie drink before each meal to keep the stomach full and decrease hunger, and then drink additional water an hour after the meal to avoid problems with digestion. If you drink sodas or juice, the high sugar content of these beverages will boost your insulin level and make you even hungrier.

Fruits and Vegetables

Fruits and vegetables are generally safe, but you must clean the skin because pesticides adhere to it. Eat fresh vegetables instead of canned vegetables. When vegetables are cooked, it should be done at low temperatures to preserve their vitamins and nutrients. Oranges and lemons are rich in vitamin C and antioxidants. Carrots and green vegetables are high in carotinoids, which are substances that protect the body from some types of cancers, such as breast and colon cancer. Tomatoes are high in lycopene, which is a potent antioxidant that protects against prostate cancer. Cauliflower and broccoli are rich in substances called isothiocyanates, which help stop the progression of toxic substances in our body, particularly the substances involved in breast and colorectal cancers.

The Magic of Olive Oil

Central to the Italian diet is the use of olive oil, which is truly a magical substance. Not only is it very flavorful, but because it is 76 percent monounsaturated fat, it is especially beneficial for your heart in helping to control the "bad" LDL (low density lipoprotein) cholesterol while raising the "good" HDL (high density lipoprotein) levels. The use of olive oil dates back over 5,000 years and was central to the civilizations of the ancient Greeks and Romans, who used it not just for cooking and eating, but also as a source of fuel and medicine.

While olive oil comes in different varieties, from extra-virgin to pure, the best is the green pomace oil, which comes from the first pressing of the olives and is the least processed. An easy way to tell if your olive oil comes from the first pressing is to look at the color. Olive oil that is green comes from the first pressing. The more processed the olive oil is, the more yellow the oil is. If you have not used olive oil before and are just beginning to learn to enjoy its delicious taste, you can add balsamic vinegar to it and use it as a salad dressing for your salad or as a delicious dip for your bread (rather than butter).

Moderate Alcohol Consumption

The consumption of any type of alcohol, including wine, before eating will increase the secretion of pancreatic enzymes and also make you hungry. Drinking wine during the meal has the same effect, but with food already in your system, the enzymes already have something to work on and the wine will not induce further hunger. I suggest drinking a glass of red wine during your meal (a five-ounce glass is equivalent to one serving) because it aids digestion by stimulating pancreatic secretion and also works to decrease bad cholesterol. Red wine is especially beneficial because, unlike white wine, it is fermented with the skin of the grapes, which contain antioxidants that help prevent blood clots and the formation of plaque in arteries.

There is a saying in Italy that wine makes good blood, "buon sangue".

Limited Red Meat

One thing that you may find striking about the Italian/ Mediterranean diet is the small amount of red meat consumed. Adults really do not need to eat red meat more than once or twice a month. On the other hand, children and adolescents need to eat more because they are growing and require more protein.

One reason to reduce your consumption of red meat is because of the correlation that has been found between animal fats and cancer. Another reason is if you have a cholesterol problem. The fat in animals provides a great vehicle for pesticides, herbicides, and fungicides used on farms. It also transports benzopyrine, which is found in large cities. How the meat is treated before it is eaten is also important. If you barbecue the meat at a very high temperature, the protein can become saturated with hydrocarbons, which are toxic.

No Food at Night

The food that we eat at night needs to be eaten at least three hours before going to bed; otherwise, it will just sit in our stomach and more readily turn into fat. I had one overweight patient who complained that she was not eating very much. She did not have anything during the day, only at night. When I asked for more details, she stated she was eating a salad around 7:00 p.m., a sandwich around 8:00, and then between 8:00 and 9:00, she would eat dessert and then go to bed. The dessert was the main cause of her weight gain because most of the food had no nutritional content and because there was no activity after eating the food.

Take a Walk After Eating

This brings us to the Italian tradition of taking a walk after dinner. A pleasant stroll keeps us active and helps burn off the calories from dinner. There is also no snacking after dinner, only a cup of herbal tea, coffee or a glass of digestive liquor. It is also good to wait two to four hours before going to bed. They eat small dinners, preferring to take their main meal at lunch.

The Necessity of Carbohydrates

Why do we talk about the importance of low-carbohydrate diets in America when carbohydrates are an integral part of the Italian diet? I think it is more out of concern for the large portions of carbohydrates that Americans consume rather than their effect. Carbohydrates are a necessary part of our diet. They fill our stomach and give us the satisfaction we need to continue dieting.

Eat Slowly

Eating your food slowly will aid digestion and enhance enjoyment, so take the time to savor the different textures and flavors of the foods you are eating. Try to begin each meal with a food that makes you feel full faster such as a green salad. What you want to avoid are the high calorie items like candy, cookies, ice cream, and cake. Later on, I will suggest some great desserts that are low in calories and fat and that you can eat as much of as you desire.

The interesting part of the Italian diet is that it includes pizza, spaghetti, and tortellini, all of which contain carbohydrates and fat.

The interesting part of the Italian diet is that it includes pizza, spaghetti, and tortellini, all of which contain carbohydrates and fat.

A Good Daily Intake

1. Breakfast is a bowl of whole-grain, low-sugar cereal, a cappuccino or café au lait and a single "biscotto" or cookie.

2. Lunch is a first dish of a small amount of soup, rice or pasta a second dish of chicken, fish, or meat, a side dish with vegetables, green salad, fresh fruit, and occasionally a small dessert

3. Dinner is not the main meal and is composed of either a first dish or a second dish and a green salad and fruit.

Italians Enjoy Their Food and Their Lives

The power of the family is truly an impressive but underestimated force.

Conversation around the house at suppertime has been shown to be a source of relaxation and contentment. People who are nervous at the table tend to eat more, particularly sweets. The contentment Italians derive from sitting down together has an immense impact on their weight and self-image. You do not have to be a model or an actor to take care of yourself. I believe that putting some effort into skin care, clothing choices, grooming, and general physical fitness will increase your motivation to lose weight.

A Pleasing Appearance

As you start losing weight and see your appearance improving, you will be better able to continue losing the pounds and keeping them off. And when you start feeling good about yourself, you gain more control of the psychological aspects that make you depressed, and this will enable you to decrease the stress that contributes to weight gain. Your thoughts and behavior are going to catch up with your new, slimmer appearance, and you will be able to enjoy your new beauty.

Having a pleasing appearance is not just for the young, but also for middle-aged people and seniors as well. In Italy, you can find women in their 50s and 60s who still have nice figures, Sophia Loren being one of the most well known.

Food as a Tranquilizer

Having a firm grasp of your body image and spending less time eating means that you will have a more balanced, stress-free life. On the other hand, people who are stressed, have a demanding job, or are depressed tend to eat more. Food can serve as a tranquilizer for people who are very depressed.

It is important to enjoy life.

Now I do not want to imply that Italians have all the answers on how to live a good life and lose weight. What I am trying to point out, however, is that as a society, Italians lead less stressful lives, enjoy a better quality of life. An Italian lifestyle is a combination of diet, physical activity, social interaction, and care of the body and soul. Italians try to be happy with everyone and everything. Focusing on sad thoughts only keeps sadness alive and prevents you from engaging in the world around you.

In the last 20 years, these cultural values, including the Italian attitudes toward food, have been challenged. Fast food restaurants, such as McDonald's, have been introduced into Italy, and more children have put pressure on their parents to take them there. As a result, in the last two years, for the first time in Italian culture, problems of pediatric obesity have become more prevalent. It is important to understand that America has been seen as an example to emulate for most of the rest of the world, including the Italians. They have tried to mirror every aspect of American life, not just in sports and quality of life, but also in the ways they eat. Unfortunately, this is beginning to have an impact on their weight and the prevalence of illnesses associated with obesity.

In Italy, I was taught the importance of beauty, good food, and social interaction. This is how I was raised. When I came to America, I learned the importance of working long hours under stressful conditions; I learned to compete and to work harder than others. This affected my quality of life, which began to deteriorate. As my lifestyle changed, I started eating late at night and became more reliant on fast food. I forgot all of the principles that I learned when I was growing up. In a little over a year, I gained 25 pounds. Only exercise and returning to the principles I had learned as a child brought my weight back down.

I believe that most college students in the United States eat unhealthy food, as I did, because healthy food is more expensive and because they do not have the time to cook. Eventually, I was able to locate the healthier foods in supermarkets and made the effort to prepare my own food.

College Years

Many of my patients have told me that they were lean when they started college, but during and immediately after college, they gained a lot of weight. College students need to learn how to survive by not eating unhealthy foods and exercising so that they do not become obese.

Alcohol is another issue on many college campuses. In Italy, children learn the pleasures and limitations of wine and alcoholic beverages at the family table; most American kids do not experience alcohol until they start college, when they do not have parental supervision. Alcohol consumption is not only a social and behavioral problem that can end up in addiction, but it contains many calories as well. I believe unhealthy food intake and excess alcohol consumption could be avoided in large part if families kept in better touch with their kids during their college years.

Power of the Family

Eating dinner with family every weekend was very enjoyable when I lived in Italy. Since coming to this country, it is one of the things I miss most. The homes of Italians represent their families and their lives together. It does not matter if a person lives in a house or in an apartment. The important thing is the warmth, the serenity and the necessity of living together, which carries a high value for Italians. Most Italian families will live and die in the same house and keep the house for generations to come. The houses are well kept and are passed from father to son or father to daughter. In the U.S., houses are more like commodities and they are sold according to job requirements that may take a person to several different cities during his or her professional career.

We must regain the pleasure of buying fresh food and cooking fresh food in order to lose weight and live a healthier lifestyle.

Cultural Differences

The cultural differences between the U.S. and Italy are reflected on both a large scale, such as the architecture of U.S. and Italian cities, and on a very small scale, such as the different sizes of U.S. and Italian refrigerators. The cities in Europe are "centripete," which means that everything is done in the city. Very few people live in villas or houses; most people live in condos or apartments near the stores, where everyone knows each other. This is true not only in the small cities, but also in the larger cities. In the United States, cities are built in "centrifuge" fashion, which means people come to the city to work, but at the end of the day, they return to their houses on the outskirts of town. It is not uncommon, particularly on the East and West coasts, to have people commuting an hour or more to work. In contrast, driving an hour in Italy means going from Venice to Verona, two cities at the opposite ends of the same region.

The structure of Italian cities allows you to meet people. Many of my friends and family would go to stores together. This would happen quite frequently, because we did not have a large refrigerator or freezer. Thus, we would have to buy bread, vegetables, and fish every day. This was not a great inconvenience because the stores were conveniently located only a block or so away from our home. Shopping for food was not just a daily necessity, but also an opportunity for social interaction among family and friends. We would often stop to chat with family and acquaintances along the way.

Refrigerators and pantries in Italy tend to be much smaller than those in the U.S. Italians prefer to shop for food on a daily basis and store only the most essential of cooking ingredients. Grocery shopping in the U.S. is done, instead, on a weekly basis and consumers opt all too often for foods with a long shelf life and preservatives so that they may later "shop" from their kitchens. What also hasn't helped is all the emphasis that U.S. kitchen designers have placed in recent years on large-scale, state-of-the-art appliances and show-stopping pantry spaces. Impressive as they may be in design and function, they haven't necessarily fostered healthier eating habits as kitchen owners have tended to fill up all the extra space with sodas, bags of snacks, canned goods or frozen foods rich in preservatives.

Life in the U.S.

While, realistically, we cannot change many of the stressful, fast-paced aspects of the lifestyle that we live here in the United States, we can learn to control the harmful effects of stress and poor diet by making some basic changes in our food consumption. Fortunately, this is becoming an easier task in America as supermarkets begin to respond to a demand for fresh, healthier foods.

Childhood Obesity:
Lifestyle is Inherited and Bequeathed

Physicians and scientists do not really know if the tendency toward weight gain is genetic or behavioral. However, at this point, we believe it is behavioral.

As I mentioned previously, it is also important to change our eating habits for the sake of our children. In general, if parents are obese, then their children are at high risk for obesity. Physicians and scientists do not really know if this tendency toward weight gain is genetic or purely behavioral. For example, obese parents almost invariably keep unhealthy food around the house; thus, because of this habit, their children learn poor eating habits. Statistics show that 80% of children born to two obese parents will become obese and that 30% of obese individuals do not engage in any physical activity.

A study recently published in the New England Journal of Medicine found an unprecedented increase in obesity at younger and younger ages and predicted that if the rapid rise in pediatric obesity continues unabated, it could actually shorten the life expectancy of our children by two to five years. This would make the current generation of children, the first to live a shorter lifespan than their parents!

Most obese people have the so called "snack often syndrome" because they eat snacks in between meals. Most of the time obesity starts with fast foods, which contain a lot of fat and carbohydrates, and are readily available.

In my practice, I see many overweight patients who bring their overweight children with them on their appointments. My advice to them is to take immediate action; big children become bigger adults and have a much harder time losing weight later in life. I have never understood parents who say, "He's young, he'll lose the weight when he gets older, and, besides, he's going to exercise." People who are overweight usually do not exercise because it is more difficult to move around or because they have health issues, such as pulmonary or heart disease, which limit vigorous activity. It is important, therefore, to keep our children in shape while they are young, so that they will learn healthy habits and maintain them throughout their lives.

Good meals are the key to a healthy lifestyle, not good snacks.

An Informal Study

A study endorsed by the Surgeon General used a pedometer, which is a small machine that looks like a beeper, to measure the number of steps children need to take during the day in order to stay healthy and maintain an appropriate body mass index (BMI). The Surgeon General suggests that young girls between six and 12 years of age need to take 12,000 steps per day, while boys need to take 15,000 steps per day.

My eight-year-old son, Edoardo, performed an interesting experiment to see if the children at his school were getting enough exercise. He wore his pedometer from the time he arrived at school until the end of the school day. He also wore the pedometer between 3:00 p.m. and 8:30 p.m. to see how much exercise he received after school. I believed that my son was very active and would easily match the recommended numbers because he rides his bike and plays basketball and soccer. Unfortunately, I was wrong. The average number of steps he was taking during the school hours of 7:30 a.m. to 3:00 p.m. was between 3,000 and 5,400. The average number of steps he was taking after school was between 3,600 and 6,700. Combining the data, he was taking an average of 7,000 to 12,000 steps per day. Edoardo's numbers were below his goal of 15,000 steps per day.

> We need to continue to enjoy the pleasure of eating while teaching our children to understand when and how we need to eat and what foods we need to eat.

From the informal study above, I realized that obesity is sometimes encouraged at school, where kids are not engaging in enough physical activity to approach the goals suggested by the Surgeon General. In addition, the vending machines and snack bars found in so many schools serve high calorie foods that do not help kids learn healthy eating habits.

We need to continue to enjoy the pleasure of eating while teaching our children to understand when and how we need to eat and what foods we need to eat.

Foods That Make Us Feel Full

High calorie foods actually worsen hunger by increasing both the acid in the stomach and the insulin in the blood.

Which foods make us feel full? Which ones make us feel hungry? Let's start with a brief discussion of how different kinds of food and drink affect the stomach and feelings of hunger. Italians sometimes drink a mixed cocktail called "aperitivo" before their meals. An aperitivo can be as simple as a glass of Prosecco or a combination of fruit juices and sweet vermouth. The alcohol in an aperitivo increases the secretion of acid in the stomach. The increased production of acid, in turn, increases hunger. Visualization of good food, as well as the smell of food, sends messages from our brain to our stomach to produce more acid and start contracting. The result is that we feel the need to eat. This process starts the production of enzymes that enable us to fully digest the food.

What Foods Make us Feel Hungry?

1) Sweets

If we eat foods high in calories, such as desserts, our hunger will not diminish. High calorie foods actually worsen hunger by increasing both the acid in the stomach and the insulin in the blood. Increased insulin makes the body want more sugar. Thus, eating sugary food can become a vicious cycle; the more sugar we eat, the more insulin we produce; the more insulin we produce, the more sugar we think we need.

2) Fried Foods

Another type of food that will increase rather than diminish hunger is fried food. Have you ever wondered why you are still hungry after you have eaten a fast food meal? French fries are one of the main culprits because fried food increases the acidity in the stomach. Because fries are "fried" and very fatty, they also increase the production of bile from our gallbladder. The contraction of the gallbladder releases bile in the small intestine, which, in turn, increases the contraction of the intestine. The contraction of the intestine increases the release of hormones involved in the digestive process, which indirectly will increase the release of insulin through hormones named incretins. We are, therefore, back to square one, feeling the urge for more and more food. If we eat boiled potatoes, this physiological process will be present but much slower.

3) Acidic Foods

What other foods will increase our urge for food? All foods that contain acid increase acidity in the stomach and contribute to hunger pangs. Excess acidity can also irritate the delicate lining of the stomach. Every time I have a patient with gastritis, ulcers, or acid reflux disease, my first suggestion to him or her is to avoid foods that increase acidity and eat pasta. These foods include coffee, mints, tomatoes, pickles, and foods high in sugar. Other foods, such as red peppers, are good for the stomach because they increase the production of a protein called Capsain, which protects our stomach.

Everything that has a crust, such as various breads, acts as an irritant to the cells of the stomach. The cells react by producing more acid. Acidity is one of the stomach's defense mechanisms. Similarly, some grilled foods, especially those that are over-grilled, will be seen by the stomach as an attack on the layer of the cells, and it will try to destroy the burned meat with increased acid production. It is important, therefore, to avoid foods that trigger higher acid production in the stomach because not only do they compromise the health of the stomach lining, but they also increase hunger.

What Foods Make Us Feel Full?

But the question we all want the answer to is what foods can we eat that will fill our stomachs while contributing to weight loss? The only foods that have been shown to fill the stomach completely, decrease acidity, and reduce hunger pangs are those containing carbohydrates.

What types and how many carbohydrates can we eat? I believe that low-carbohydrate diets have a role in weight loss. However, the main reason carbohydrates have gotten such a bad reputation is because of the quantity of these foods that are being eaten. When you eat pasta in a restaurant, for example, the portion sizes are so large that one portion would be considered four portions in Italy!

How do carbohydrates work? If we eat the crust on a piece of bread, the crust increases the acidity of the stomach. Toasted bread and bagels invariably increase the acidity of the stomach, yet they are one of the most common breakfasts in America. Butter increases the contraction of the stomach; therefore, after one hour, we feel hungry again. A much better alternative is to eat the bagel with cream cheese because the cheese absorbs the acid, thereby decreasing hunger.

The only foods that have been shown to fill the stomach completely, decrease acidity, and reduce hunger pangs are those containing carbohydrates.

Fresh cheeses and pasta, especially in combination, are good for the stomach because they decrease acidity and decrease any feelings of being hungry after you finish a meal.

Pasta and cheese are good companion foods, because the pasta buffers the acid from the cheese. Fresh cheese is better than seasoned cheese. If you eat Parmigiano cheese that has been seasoned, it will increase acidity, but this acidity is then absorbed by the pasta. The Italians use this combination of foods in many of their dishes.

It is important to remember that carbohydrates are not bad in and of themselves. They play a very positive role in absorbing acid in the stomach. However, it is a mistake to live completely on a carbohydrate-free diet. In fact, it is almost impossible. Carbohydrates are found not just in pasta and cereals. Fruits and vegetables also bring carbohydrates into the body. How does that happen? Grapes and honeydew melons are full of a sugar called fructose. The fructose is absorbed in our intestine. It passes from the intestine into the liver, where an enzyme turns the fructose into glucose.

In the liver, the glucose is either sent to the rest of the body or stored. If our body needs the glucose, the sugar goes directly to the cells that need the glucose, and it will be burned for energy. If we do not need the glucose, the liver stores it so it can be used at another time. When too much glucose is stored, it turns into fat chains. Therefore, every food containing carbohydrates that is eaten in excess can form fat cells.

There are some carbohydrates, such as rice, that have many healthy properties. When I was growing up in Italy, we ate rice mixed with a small amount of olive oil, or we boiled the rice and ate it in the water in which it was boiled. We did this because the water contains maltose, another sugar contained in rice, and the maltose coats the cells of the stomach, thereby decreasing the production of acid. If you have gastritis, it works better than some anti-acid medicines!

Whether carbohydrates are a good or bad part of our diet depends on how they are used in our meals.

Foods That Make Us Feel Full

Pasta (with oil, fresh cheese, or a light tomato sauce - too much tomato is BAD).

Baked potato (no toppings).

Well-boiled rice with few condiments because the use of condiments, sauces, and dips can increase your appetite.

Reasons We Overeat

While no weight-loss book can solve all the psychological issues surrounding food, we can directly address the physiological feeling of hunger which motivates so much overeating. And if we can find a way to feel full while dieting, we will be better able to lose weight and cope with the other issues surrounding food, many of which can be quite complex.

The Main Reasons We Tend to Overeat

We like food, and we like to eat.

We like a particular food, so we eat more of it.

We eat because we are going to meetings that are often conducted over lunch or dinner.

We eat because we are depressed.

We do not eat in public because we do not want to attract attention to ourselves. However, we eat more in the privacy of our home instead.

We eat because we want to try a different experience.

We eat because we never feel full.

There seems to exist an endless list of reasons to eat: people eat when they are stressed, sad, lonely, bored, tired, or, sometimes, when they crave a certain food without really being hungry. These non-physiological factors can be dangerous. Uncontrolled, they can lead to many extra pounds in just a few short months.

Some foods really do act to elevate mood or create a sense of calm. Chocolate, particularly dark chocolate, contains a protein called tyramine, which increases the production of the neurotransmitter, serotonin. Serotonin promotes happiness and serenity. Therefore, chocolate can be a good food if consumed sensibly. The average American, however, eats 12 pounds of chocolate in a year! It is far better to purchase a high quality dark chocolate to eat in small amounts than to consume large quantities of a cheaper but inferior quality of chocolate that leaves you feeling unsatisfied.

There is a seemingly endless list of reasons to eat.

Carbohydrates are another food that produces a sense of well-being. Like chocolate, carbohydrates increase the production of serotonin, which regulates sleep, mood, food intake, and pain tolerance. Anti-depressants such as Prozac, Zoloft and other drugs work in the same fashion.

Some foods really do act to elevate mood or create a sense of calm.

There is no problem with consuming foods that promote a sense of well-being as long as they are consumed in moderation. The question is not whether you can live without chocolate or whether you can live without pasta. The question is: Can you eat the food you enjoy in small quantities? It is important to understand that you cannot live completely without these foods and that there are days when you should eat them. I do not know many Italians who can live without pasta.

I first met my wife and her family, who are originally Italian, in Pittsburgh, Pennsylvania. The first thing that struck me about my father-in-law was his love of pasta. He had to eat it at least once or twice a day. He often said that no meal was complete without a course of pasta.

A Successful Eating Program Includes:

1. Understanding some of the reasons you overeat,
2. Controlling portion sizes,
3. Finding ways to make your body feel full, so that you can lose weight without feelings of hunger or deprivation.

Lowering Calories to Lose Weight

Lowering the number of calories consumed is essential to losing weight, pure and simple. Calories are the basic measurement of the energy stored in food. One food calorie is the amount of energy needed to raise one kilo or 2.2 pounds of water one degree Centigrade. There is no difference between a fat calorie, a carbohydrate calorie, and a protein calorie; all contain exactly the same amount of energy. The digestive process serves to release the energy in food so the body can move, see, think, breathe, speak, and perform all its other amazing functions. Any unused energy is stored as body fat.

To stay slim and healthy, we need to balance the energy input with the energy output.

It is important to remember that different types of food vary widely in the number of calories they contain. A bite of chocolate has many more calories than a bite of lettuce. This is one reason a balanced diet is vital. By filling your stomach with lower calorie food, you will gain less weight. A permanent change to healthy eating patterns and food choices will automatically decrease your caloric intake and help you achieve an optimum weight. Once this change is in place, you will not need to think about calories as much as you must do when you are first starting to lose weight.

If you know how many carbohydrate, protein, fat, and alcohol products you consume, you can calculate your caloric intake for the day. The average number of calories contained in these food categories per gram is illustrated in the table below:

Carbohydrate	4 calories★
Fat	9 calories★
Alcohol	7 calories★

★ per gram

When counting calories in your food, you should include everything: the butter you put on your bread, the dressing on your salad, and the M & M's that you grabbed from your friend's desk.

How Many Calories Do You Need?

An average 25-year-old needs approximately 2,400 calories to maintain his or her weight. After age 25, you should decrease your caloric intake by 2% every ten years. So if you are 35, you need 2,350 calories, and so forth. Also men usually consume about 10% more calories than women because they have 10% to 20% more muscle mass.

A good guideline is to use the "percentage" rule. It provides a safe and healthy way to lose weight. First, you need to figure out the average number of calories you eat now. For instance, suppose you consume 3,000 calories a day and would like to lose 20 pounds.

First, convert the pounds into a percentage:
> 20 pounds becomes 20%

Then perform the following calculation:
> 3,000 calories x 20% = 3,000 x .20 = 600 calories.

Then you do the subtraction:
> 3,000 calories − 600 calories = 2,400 calories.

Thus, if you want to lose 20 pounds, you should reduce your caloric intake to 2,400 calories per day. By following this rule, you can lose between ½ to 1 pound per week. It will take approximately 6 to 8 months to lose this weight. If you want to lose more weight, you must reduce the amount of calories you consume even further. The calorie table in Appendix 1 will help you to calculate the calories in various foods.

The Food and Drug Administration (FDA) Guidelines for the Labeling of Foods

A low calorie food is one that contains 120 calories or less per 100 grams (about 2½ ounces).

Low fat means that there are 2 grams of fat per 100 grams.

Low cholesterol means that the item contains less than 20 mg. of cholesterol per 100 grams, with no more than 2 grams of saturated fat.

Low sodium means that the food contains 140 mg. or less of sodium per 100 grams.

Light means that the food item is low in fat and calories.

Healthy means that there are key nutrients such as vitamins, calcium, protein, fiber, etc.

The Food Pyramid and Daily Servings

Recently, the U.S. Department of Agriculture (USDA) updated its Food Guide Pyramid to reflect new knowledge about health and nutrition. I find it a bit complicated! I think the old pyramid provides a more comprehensive guide to making healthier food choices and to stress the importance of drinking plenty of water and engaging in daily exercise.

Please look at the pyramid on the next page. The pyramid shape shows which foods you should eat more or less of. Red meat, and foods high in saturated animal fats like butter, should be eaten sparingly, while those at the bottom, such as whole grains and vegetables, should be eaten more frequently. To lose weight and maintain health, you should focus on eating foods from the lower portion of the pyramid.

Controlling the amount of food you consume will help you control your caloric intake. You will need to get used to thinking of foods in terms of portion or serving sizes. What constitutes a serving? Different foods, even if they are found on a single plate, make up different servings.

When choosing foods, you should keep in mind that they often come in different sizes. For example, bagels often come in small or large sizes; a large bagel with cream cheese is considered to be almost two servings. At the end of this chapter is a list of foods considered to be a single serving. Study this chart and refer to it because the portions are smaller than most Americans consume. For example one serving of bread is one slice of bread. Half a cup of pasta is one serving—and not the plateful that most restaurants serve. At mealtimes, try not to eat pasta, beans, and potatoes together because they are basically the same type of food.

When shopping at the supermarket, be sure to examine the food labels on the packages of the food you are buying. Under the Nutrition Facts sections of the label, you will see listed the number of calories per serving, as well as the amounts of fat, cholesterol, and sodium per serving. The chart on page 43 outlines the number of servings you should be consuming for a total intake of 1,500 and 1,800 calories per day, if you would like to lose weight.

> You will need to get used to thinking of foods in terms of portions or serving sizes.

The Modified Pyramid

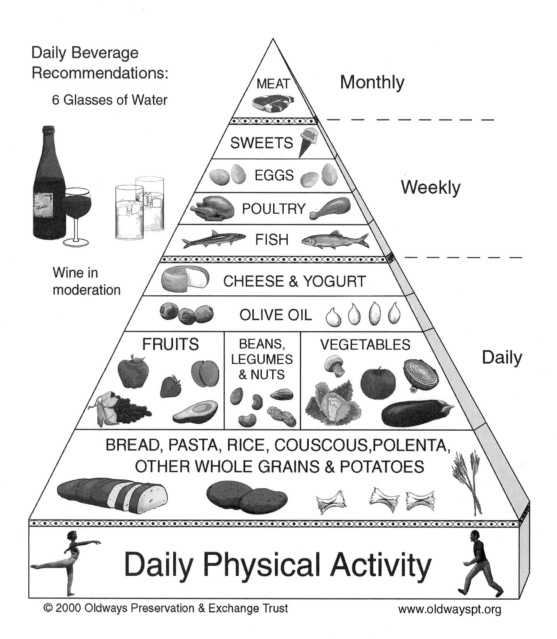

Daily Beverage
Recommendations:

6 Glasses of Water

Wine in
moderation

MEAT — Monthly

SWEETS

EGGS

POULTRY — Weekly

FISH

CHEESE & YOGURT

OLIVE OIL

FRUITS | BEANS, LEGUMES & NUTS | VEGETABLES — Daily

BREAD, PASTA, RICE, COUSCOUS, POLENTA, OTHER WHOLE GRAINS & POTATOES

Daily Physical Activity

Suggested Number of Servings per Day by Food Group

Calories	Bread	Vegetable	Fruit	Milk	Meat
1500	6	3	3	6	6 ounces of cooked meat
1800	8	5	4	8	7 ounces of cooked meat

Breads, Pasta, Rice and Potatoes

½ cup cooked cereal, rice, or pasta

1 ounce hot cereal, uncooked

½ hamburger bun or English muffin

1 small roll, biscuit, or muffin

1 slice of bread

4-inch pizza bread, white or wheat

3 medium bread sticks, about ¼ inch thick and 4¾ inches long

½ cup pasta

1 medium baked potato

½ cup potato salad

10 French fries

¾ cup sweet potatoes

5 to 6 small or 3 to 4 large crackers

9 animal crackers

2 pretzels

2 4" rice or popcorn cakes

3 cups of popcorn (fat-free)

1-7" flour tortilla

1-7" corn tortilla

12 tortilla chips

2 6" corn taco shells

Fruit

1 medium apple, banana, or orange

3 medium apricots

2 dried apricots

4 canned apricots, drained

½ cup blueberries

11 cherries

½ cup sweetened canned cherries

½ cup chopped fresh, cooked or canned fruit in juice

13 grapes

½ large grapefruit

1 large kiwi fruit

½ medium mango

1/8 of a medium melon

7 melon balls

½ medium papaya

1½ medium plums

½ cup raspberries

½ cup strawberries

½ cup berries

½ cup fruit salad

¾ cup fruit juice

½ cup dried fruit

Each of the portions is considered to be one serving

Vegetables

1 artichoke

3 stems of broccoli

4 medium Brussels sprouts

7-8 baby carrots

1 7" celery stick

½ cup coleslaw

10 medium green onions

1 cup mixed green salad

½ cup leafy cooked greens

1 medium green or red pepper

1 medium ear of corn

7 medium mushrooms

8 fresh onion rings

9 snow peas

15 medium radishes

9 green peas

6 slices of yellow summer squash or zucchini

1 medium tomato

5 cherry tomatoes

½ cup tomatoes or spaghetti sauce

½ cup vegetable juice

1 cup vegetable soup

½ cup cooked vegetables

½ cup chopped, raw vegetables

Beans and Nuts

1 cup bean soup

½ cup cooked beans, peas, or other legumes

2 tablespoons peanut butter

Eggs

1 yolk and one egg white

2 egg whites

Dairy

1 cup milk or buttermilk

½ cup dried, non-fat milk

½ cup evaporated milk

1½ ounces of natural cheeses

2 ounces of processed cheese

½ cup cottage cheese

¼ cup ricotta cheese

1 cup yogurt

1 cup frozen yogurt

White Meat and Fish

2 to 3 ounces of cooked poultry, without skin or bones

2 to 3 ounces of cooked fish, without bones

2 to 3 ounces of drained, canned fish

1 turkey frankfurter

1 ounce of lean turkey ham or bacon

6 medium shrimp

9 oysters

Red Meat

2 to 3 ounces of cooked lean beef, pork, or lamb without bones

1 beef or pork frankfurter

1 ounce of lean ham or Canadian bacon

Sweets

1/16 of a two-layer cake, without frosting

1/5 of a 10-inch angel food cake

Miscellaneous

5 ounces of wine

12 ounces of beer

1½ ounces of 80 proof alcohol

Hidden Calories and Holiday Feasts

Having just a bagel or muffin at breakfast may sound innocent. Unfortunately, the size of many breakfast foods has tripled in recent years and now we have muffins the size of softballs and six-inch bagels instead of the original four-inch bagels. As a consequence, the calorie counts have also risen exponentially. For example:

· Muffins. These can have as many as 590 calories and 24 grams of fat. The reduced-fat blueberry muffin can pack 450 calories.

· Bagels. A traditionally-sized bagel has about 200-300 calories. A large bagel might have double the calories.

· Salads. The majority of salad dressings and toppings contributes significantly to the amount of needless calories.

Beverages

Some beverages are extremely caloric. A 12-ounce can of regular beer contains 146 calories. A liqueur might have 186 calories. A 3-ounce glass of wine has an average of 72 calories. Clearly, alcohol should be consumed in moderation if you want to lose weight. One glass of wine is beneficial because it helps decrease cholesterol. A bottle of wine, however, contains far too many calories.

A large Frappuccino with whipped cream contains around 710 calories and 26 grams of fat. A large coffee with whipped cream contains 490 calories with 26 grams of fat. If you can't do without a daily cup of gourmet coffee, compromise by doing the following:

1) Ask for skim milk.

2) Skip the whipped cream on top and any caloric flavoring (especially coconut cream).

3) Order a smaller size.

By applying these rules, you can trim down your coffee to 170 calories and 1.5 grams of fat!

Holiday Feasts

Holiday feasts are especially notorious for their excessive calories. Since gravy, pumpkin pie and other dishes are not typically Italian, we took some of the following ideas from holiday feast web pages. Gravy, for example, is often viewed as a harmless topping for turkey, but three to four ladles of this substance actually carry a staggering 400 calories!

It is important to gain control of hidden calorie consumption.

Stopping at the vending machine could cost you more calories than lunch if you're not careful.

The chart below offers a realistic breakdown of the calories hidden in a typical holiday feast. The meal is modified from various food website resources.

A Realistic Portrayal of a Typical Holiday Feast

	Calories	Grams of Fat
Appetizers:		
1 cup mixed nuts	795	74.0
5 celery sticks with cream cheese	225	21.2
10 crackers with cream cheese	705	48.9
Main Meal:		
8 oz. white and dark turkey meat	480	13.8
1 cup mashed potatoes	305	19.0
1 cup stuffing	595	56.5
3-4 ladles of gravy	400	36
½ cup green beans	50	–
½ cup candied sweet potatoes	300	6.0
½ cup cranberry sauce	209	trace
2 rolls with butter	180	22.0
1 slice pecan pie	360	31.8
1 cup coffee with cream and sugar	50	–
1 glass of cider or wine	150	0
Totals	4,804 calories	329.2 grams of fat

"That's OK," you may say, "I'll just run an extra mile tomorrow."

Well, if you are planning to run off all the calories from this meal, you will need to allow for about 10 hours.

This feast carries a grand total of 4,804 calories and 329 grams of fat. And that's before you start on the leftovers on the following days. Now, granted, this is a lot of food, but my point is that most people underestimate how much they eat, especially during the holidays. Now let's try lightening up this meal and see what happens to the numbers.

A Lightened Holiday Feast

	Calories	Grams of Fat
Appetizers:		
1 cup tomato juice	50	0.0
5 celery sticks with low-fat cream cheese	78	5.0
5 reduced-fat wheat crackers with low-fat cream cheese	131	3.9
Main Meal:		
8 oz. roasted white turkey meat with no skin	193	5.6
1 cup mashed potatoes with evaporated skim milk	62	1.2
1 cup stuffing made with non-fat chicken broth	221	5.8
¼ cup turkey gravy	25	trace
½ cup baby carrots	31	1.3-
½ cup green beans	46	trace
baked sweet potatoes with margarine	235	4.1
¼ cup cranberry sauce	180	trace
2 whole grain rolls	180	2.0
1 slice low-fat pumpkin pie	230	trace
1 cup coffee with evaporated skim milk	27	0
1 glass of champagne	175	0
Totals	1,864 calories	26.3 grams of fat

As you can see, this dinner is only 1,864 calories and has just 26.3 grams of fat—a big difference!

Turning Around Your Thanksgiving Meal

How can you create low-fat versions of your traditional Thanksgiving recipes? The goal is to lower calories without sacrificing the delicious taste.

Recipe Makeover Techniques

Please use evaporated skim milk, fat-free chicken broth, or egg substitute. Avoid heavy sauces or gravies. You can also replace sugar with a sugar substitute.

Turkey and Stuffing

Foods **do not** have to be loaded with calories and fat to taste good.

- Pick a turkey that is not self-basting. This way you can control the amount of fat added while cooking.
- Roast the turkey on a rack, so the fat drips away.
- When carving, remove the skin, because this is where a lot of the fat is.
- Use a fat separator for the roasting pan juices.
- Use a dry package of turkey gravy mix for added flavor and thickening.
- Don't stuff the turkey with dressing as it absorbs much of the fat. Bake your stuffing in a casserole dish.
- In the corn bread for the stuffing, use applesauce in place of oil.
- Sauté onions and celery in a small amount of olive oil. You can also soften your celery and onions by cooking them in a small amount of chicken broth which can be used also to add additional moisture.

Tips for the Holiday Season

- Decide ahead of time how you will handle social pressure ("No, thank you, I am full.").
- Share one dessert with a friend, limit the serving size, or scrape off the high-fat whipped cream topping.
- Volunteer to bring a favorite low-sugar dessert, such as plain cookies, baked apples, or sugar-free pudding.
- This is not the time to take a holiday from your daily exercise routine. Continue your workouts in addition to engaging in extra activities, such as parking far from the mall or even walking to the mall. Power walk while shopping.
- Don't feel pressured to finish everthing on your plate.

Vegetables

- Serve vegetables that are steamed, grilled, or baked with a little added fat, such as margarine, or good olive oil.

- Use pineapple and/or orange juice thickened with cornstarch as a glaze for carrots or sweet potatoes.

- Bake sweet potatoes with a light touch of margarine and a sprinkle of cinnamon on top only.

- Cook carrots and green beans in fat-free chicken broth.

- Serve hot vegetables with fresh rosemary, basil, dill, or chopped sweet red pepper. Eliminate the butter.

- Use low-fat canned cream soup for cooking your vegetable casserole.

- Instead of serving vegetables with a cream or cheese sauce, top the dish with a small amount of Parmigiano Reggiano cheese and then run the dish under the broiler for a minute.

Pumpkin Pie

- Replace the eggs with an egg substitute.

- Use evaporated or skim milk.

- Use half the amount of the sugar stated in the recipe and slightly increase the spices.

- Use a light or fat-free whipped topping.

Desserts

- Cut the sugar by one-third to one-half and increase the sweet-tasting spices. Replace sugar with a sugar substitute.

- In baked goods, use applesauce instead of oil.

- Use the sugar-free, fat-free instant puddings.

- Use low-carb or fat-free whipped toppings and ice creams.

Tips during the Meal

- Eat only your favorite things. Pass up the rest. If you have to take something in order to not offend the chef, take a small amount and then don't eat it— spread it around on your plate to look as if you ate some, and only a little was left.
- Don't feel you have to clean your plate.
- Begin the meal with a salad. You'll eat less during the meal.
- Skip the rolls and bread if possible. If you must have a roll, eat a whole grain one. Whole grain rolls add fiber and nutrients; white rolls are just empty calories.
- Choose only one dessert. Enjoy it without feeling guilty! Eat the filling of a piece of pie and just a bit of the crust.
- Don't skip meals before the big meal that day. You'll be too hungry and may overeat. Treat the holiday as a regular day—three meals and a snack.

After your meal, enjoy a relaxing walk around the neighborhood.

Good and Bad Foods

Our food choices can have an enormous impact on the number of calories we consume.

Our goal in changing our eating patterns is to maximize the healthful benefits of food while minimizing calories, especially those found in carbohydrates and fat. Low-carbohydrate diets have been very popular lately, because a lot of excess weight comes from ingesting too many carbohydrates. When we gain weight, there may be an impairment of the hormone, insulin, which helps process our food intake, particularly in regard to fats and sugars. When there is insulin dysfunction or insulin resistance—a common occurrence in obese patients—there is increased fat storage. It is very important, therefore, for dieters to keep their carbohydrate intake under control. It is also important to distinguish between good and bad carbohydrates because not all carbohydrates are bad.

Bad Carbohydrates

The bad carbohydrates are those found in baked goods, such as pastries, cookies, cakes, and most of the industrially-made white breads, particularly when they do not have any fiber. Candy and other sweets tend to be high in refined white sugar, another bad carbohydrate. When you read the labels on food packages, you will note that sugar comes in many guises, such as corn sweeteners, fructose, glucose, dextrose, lactose, and maltose.

Many of us have been told that carbohydrates are less fattening than fat, but in practice, this is not always true. Fat or butter gives a satiety effect i.e. fat in fresh cheese is more slowly digested than fat in cooked or fried food. As a result, we stop eating. Refined carbohydrates, on the other hand, cause rapid changes in blood sugar levels and stimulate

The Food and Drug Administration (FDA) suggests:

Substitute	Saves Calories
1 medium sweet potato instead of 1 medium white potato	100
3 ounces ground turkey meat instead of 3 ounces ground beef	100
1 tablespoon low-fat mayonnaise vs. 1 tablespoon regular mayonnaise	85
10 small tortilla chips vs. 10 large tortilla chips	20
1 cup fat-free or 1% milk instead of 1 cup whole milk	64
1 flour tortilla instead of 1 corn tortilla	50
1 serving cottage cheese vs. 1 cup Ricotta cheese	268
2 egg whites instead of a whole egg	46
½ cup fat-free milk instead of ½ cup cream	145
½ cup regular ice cream instead of ½ cup of premium ice cream	100
2½ ounces of tuna in water instead of 2½ ounces of tuna in oil	80
½ cup fruit in juice instead of ½ cup fruit in syrup	25

further hunger, thereby encouraging overeating and obesity.

When you eliminate bad carbohydrates from your diet, insulin works more efficiently, allowing both the fat and carbohydrates we ingest to be better metabolized. If we do not eat too many carbohydrates, our body adapts to a lower intake, and cravings for carbohydrates diminish.

Good Carbohydrates

What are the good carbohydrates? Fiber-rich foods like whole grain breads, high-fiber cereals, and whole wheat pasta are good, as are fruits and vegetables. Some vegetables are better than others, especially the green-leafed varieties such as Romaine lettuce and endive. Highly colored vegetables, such as corn and carrots, contain a large percentage of carbohydrates. Tomatoes are the only highly-colored vegetable that are an exception to the rule. They do not have carbohydrates, although some of them do have a high content of sugar, which can turn into carbohydrates. On the whole, however, the benefits of eating vegetables and fruits outweigh the drawbacks.

Good Fats Versus Bad Fats

Americans tend to eat far too many high-fat foods. This is why, when you visit your doctor, you are likely to have your LDL (low-density lipoprotein) and HDL (high-density lipoprotein) cholesterol levels measured to assess your risk for heart disease. Ideally, your LDL level should be 100 mg/dl (milligrams per deciliter) or less. LDL, known as the "bad" cholesterol, increases the likelihood that plaque will build up along the interior walls of your arteries, thereby increasing your risk of a stroke or a heart attack. HDL is the "clean-up" cholesterol or "good" cholesterol, which has been shown to offer protection against heart disease. Low HDL levels, less than 35 mg/dl, increase your risk of heart disease.

As a rule, you want to avoid high-fat foods, especially those that carry the bad fats that increase your LDL levels. How do you know which are good fats versus bad fats? Saturated fats that are found in butter, lard, dairy products, meat and poultry, palm oil, kernel oil, and coconut oil increase your LDL levels and should be avoided or minimized. Unsaturated

Cooking Food Wisely

Remember that when you fry foods, the caloric intake increases dramatically. Grilling or baking food limits calories. When you do fry or sauté, however, use vegetable oil instead of butter to alleviate caloric intake. Butter is acceptable in moderate amounts. Margarine should be avoided, not because of its carbohydrate content, but because it is usually made with trans fats (hydrogenated oils), that can be a serious health hazard. Some supermarkets or health-food stores do carry a non-hydrogenated margarine.

and monounsaturated fats are preferable and have important health attributes. Unsaturated fats are found in corn, fish, sunflower, sesame, and soybean oils. Monounsaturated fats are found in canola, olive, and peanut oils.

Monounsaturated fat, an omega-3 polyunsaturated fat, is one of the best oils we can use. The tastiest oil, which contains the same omega-3 polyunsaturated fat, is olive oil. We want a diet that will lower the bad fats circulating in our bloodstream, including triglycerides and LDL, while raising our HDL levels.

Meat and Fish

Many popular diets, like the Atkins diet, recommend increasing the amounts of fat and protein you eat while reducing your carbohydrate intake. But is it really healthy to eat a diet rich in bacon or cheeseburgers? Exaggerated amounts of fat and cholesterol will eventually impair heart function.

A better strategy is to eat meat in moderation. For meats such as beef, pork, veal, and lamb stick to the leaner cuts. Chicken, turkey, and fish are inherently low in fat and are highly recommended. Fish such as trout, salmon, tuna, mackerel, bass, cod, and all white meat fish are an excellent source of omega-3 fatty acids and help promote healthy HDL levels. Squid and octopus are also very good. You should limit your intake of shellfish because most shellfish, including crab and lobster, are high in cholesterol.

Acceptable Meats and Fish

Bacon*	Beef
Chicken	Clams
Cornish hen	Crabmeat
Flounder	Ham*
Hard-boiled eggs	Herring
Lamb	Lobster
Mussels**	Omelets
Oysters**	Pork
Quail	Salmon
Sardines	Scrambled eggs
Shrimp	Soft-boiled eggs
Sole	Squid
Trout	Tuna
Turkey	Veal

*Processed meats, such as ham, bacon, pepperoni, salami, hot dogs and other luncheon meats, as well as some fish, may be cured with added sugar and will contribute extra calories and carbohydrates.

**Oysters and mussels are higher in cholesterol than other shellfish, so limit them to four ounces per day.

Eggs

What about eggs? Egg yolks have a high cholesterol content. However, they also provide a lot of natural vitamin A and E which can help keep good and bad cholesterol in balance.

Dairy

Dairy products are good for you because they have a lot of protein. Low-fat dairy products are preferable because they provide a good nutritional intake, low carbohydrates, and a normal to low amount of cholesterol.

Fruit

Not all fruit is good. In fact, some people eat too much fruit. For example, eating more than 20 grapes or several slices of watermelon or honeydew can be fattening because the sugar content is very high. Bananas have a high content of calories per gram (90 calories/gram). Adults should, therefore, limit their consumption. Tropical fruits, such as pineapples and mangos, are very sugary and cause blood glucose levels to rise rapidly.

What fruits can we eat? Strawberries, blueberries, and raspberries are excellent. These offer the lowest increase in blood sugar after consumption.

Fast Foods

Contrary to popular belief, it is not always bad to have a cheeseburger and fries. It depends on how the cheeseburger is prepared and how many fries you eat. Choose cheeseburgers with whole-wheat bread instead of white. Avoid mayonnaise and ketchup. These condiments can be much worse than the cheeseburger and fries! Use salsa or mustard instead. They are low in calories and carbohydrates.

Peanut butter and jelly sandwiches are fine, if eaten in moderation. A well-cooked pizza with tomatoes, peppers, onions, and olives is good and filling.

Condiments

Condiments can add a lot of flavor to your food without adding calories. These condiments are low in fat and low calorie:

chili powder	horseradish	hot sauce
mustard	salsa	vinegar

Burger and Fries? Limit your use of fatty mayonnaise and sugary ketchup. These condiments can be much worse than the burger or fries themselves.

Salty Foods: Foods High in Sodium

Foods high in sodium, such as potato chips and French fries, should be used in moderation. Eating too much sodium tends to increase blood pressure and also causes us to retain water, which causes weight gain.

Artificial Sweeteners

1) Sweet'n'Low™ (saccharin)

Sweet'n'Low™ (saccharin) can be safely consumed in moderation, meaning no more than three packets a day.

The effects of saccharin have been extensively studied. Scientists concluded that, in lab rats, saccharin is harmful only in extremely high doses. The Food and Drug Administration (FDA) has, therefore, removed saccharin from its list of carcinogens, basing its decision upon a thorough review of the medical literature and the National Institute of Science's statement that there is "no clear association between saccharin and human cancer." You can safely consume saccharin in moderation, meaning no more than three packets a day. One packet contains one gram of granulate sugar substitute.

2) Equal™ (aspartame)

Aspartame has also been determined safe by the United States Food and Drug Administration (FDA) and other scientific authorities. More than 200 scientific studies have confirmed its safety. Aspartame is consumed by over 2 million people around the world and is found in more than 6,000 products. Aspartame can also be used in recipes for cooking and baking. It has a clean, sweet taste, which might provide many benefits including weight control.

Equal™ (aspartame) is safe and not unsafe, as was initially reported.

A report from the Canadian Journal of Diabetes noted that aspartame is safe. Further confirmation came from a study in several human sub-populations including healthy infant children, adolescents and adults, individuals with or without diabetes, lactating women and individuals with phenylketonuria (PKU) who have a decreased ability to metabolize phenylalamine.

Another article appeared in October 2004 in the British Medical Journal confirmed that aspartame is safe and not unsafe, as was initially reported.

3) Splenda™ (sucralose)

Sucralose is an artificial sweetener that is now being sold under the name "Splenda". As reported by Dr. Joseph Mercola of mercola.com, there have only been six human trials with Splenda™. He reported that of these six trials, only two of the trials were completed and published before FDA approved sucralose for human consumption.

Splenda has taken over the sweetener industry. It has become the nation's number one selling artificial sweetener in a very short period of time. This happened between 2000 and 2004. The percentage of U.S. households using Splenda products grew from 3% to 20%. Splenda's sales reached $177 million compared to $62 million spent on aspartame-based and $50 million on saccharin-based products. Following FDA approval, a human toxicity trial was documented that lasted only three months. At that time no studies had ever been performed on children or pregnant women.

There is no question that sucralose started off as a sugar molecule. Sucralose is a synthetic chemical that was originally manufactured in a laboratory. Sucrose is a molecule, disaccharide, that contains two single sugars banded together, glucose and fructose. The chemical process to make sucralose alters the chemical composition of the sugar so much that it is converted to a chlorinate fructose. This type of sugar molecule does not occur in nature; therefore, your body does not possess the ability to metabolize it properly. As a result of this unique biochemical makeup, Splenda™ is not digested or

Because so few studies have been conducted on Splenda™ (sucralose), it might be wise to consume this sugar substitute in moderation.

Warning!

Be careful when you choose low-fat foods because low fat does not necessarily mean low calorie. In fact, the amount of carbohydrates tends to be much higher in products marked "low-fat" foods. Carbohydrates are used up very quickly by the body and causes your insulin level to go up quickly. Your body will then require more food to satisfy the insulin requirement. The following chart offers examples of low-fat foods that are not necessarily low in calories:

	Calories		Calories
8 ounces whole milk	150	8 ounces fat-free milk	85
2 tablespoons peanut butter	200	reduced fat peanut butter	190
2 tablespoons low-fat whipped topping	25	light whipped topping	20
½ cup vanilla ice cream	135	½ cup vanilla ice milk	90
½ cup beans	100	fat-free refried beans	100
Low-fat yogurt	155	non-fat yogurt	135
fig bars	110	fat-free figs bars	100
1/2 cup of 4% cottage cheese	110	1/2 cup of 1% fat cottage cheese	82

metabolized by the body; therefore, it has zero calories. If you look at the research, you will see that in fact an average of 15% of sucralose is absorbed into your digestive system and alternatively stored in your body.

One packet of Splenda™ contains one gram of dextrose, maltodextrin, sucralose.

Sodas

Regular sodas contain many carbohydrates. A can of Mountain Dew, for example, is comparable to eating a Snickers® bar, so be careful!

Carbonated drinks, drinks that bubble, like beer or sodas, can dilate the stomach and create a slower digestion with a sustained insulin level; this, in turn, could create more need for food and fat to accumulate.

Beer

Beer is high in maltose, which is a sugar that goes directly into the bloodstream and increases your insulin level. The sugar in beer turns into carbohydrates. Beer plus the carbohydrates in pizza are a powerful caloric combination, so try to drink only one beer.

Red wine is a good alternative to beer as long as it is consumed in moderation. Limit your intake to one glass per meal.

Nuts

One thing that I found interesting during my search for a good diet was the benefits of peanuts and other nuts because they have a high protein content, but not many carbohydrates. Nuts have also been shown to be a good source of fiber, as well as vitamin E, potassium, magnesium, and folic acid. You may have heard that nuts are high in fat, but unlike the animal fats found in meat, the fats found in nuts are polyunsaturated and actually benefit heart health. Walnuts are especially beneficial because they are high in alpha-linoleic acid, which is an omega-3 fatty acid that is very good for the heart.

A Nurses' Health Study that followed 86,016 women over a period of 14 years, showed that those who ate five or more ounces of nuts per week reduced their risk of cardiac death by 35 percent. Nuts should be consumed in moderation, however, because they are relatively high in calories.

Herbs

Adding herbs to your dishes is a delicious way of adding flavor without adding calories. The following herbs are all very savory:

Basil	Cayenne pepper	Cilantro
Dill	Garlic	Ginger
Oregano	Pepper	Rosemary
Sage	Tarragon	Thyme

Eliminating unhealthy foods from your diet does not mean that you have to eat unappetizing foods. What makes the modified Italian diet ideal is that it is full of healthy mono and polyunsaturated fats, such as those found in olives and olive oil, fresh fruits and vegetables, lean meat and fish, natural cheeses, and good carbohydrates. Fresh spices are also used to make food extremely flavorful.

The Italian Kitchen

To inspire nutritious cooking habits, stock your kitchen—as the Italians do—with the following items:

Dry pasta in various sizes and shapes

Rice and polenta

Extra-virgin olive oil

Balsamic vinegar

Fresh garlic cloves

Fresh basil

Fresh Italian or "flat-leafed" parsley

Rosemary (fresh or dried)

Fresh sage

Oregano (fresh or dried)

Cannellini or other types of beans (canned or dried)

Parmigiano Reggiano and fresh Italian cheeses such as mozzarella or ricotta

Fresh fruits

Fresh garden tomatoes or a good variety of canned plum tomatoes

Fresh vegetables, especially green ones

Fresh fish

Lean cuts of meat

Wine for cooking and as an accompaniment to some meals

Know Your Vegetables

As I mentioned in the previous chapter, some vegetables are better than others in terms of the amounts of carbohydrates they contain. Knowing which vegetables are low in carbohydrates will help you lose weight, especially during the first critical weeks of a diet when you are learning to restrict your caloric intake.

The list below divides popular vegetables into three categories: High, medium and low carbohydrate levels. Restrict your intake of the first to no more than one cup per day. Measure them raw to estimate the correct carbohydrate count.

High Carbohydrate Levels	Medium Carbohydrate Levels	Lower Carbohydrate Levels
1 serving (one small plate) per day is permitted	1 serving (one small plate) per day is permitted	3 servings per day are permitted
Artichoke hearts	Asparagus green	Arugula
Asparagus, white	Beet greens	Bok choy
Avocado	Broccoli rabe	Celery
Bamboo shoots	Chicory	Celery root
Bean sprouts	Cucumber	Chives
Beans	Dandelion	Endive
Beet greens	Eggplant	Escarole
Broccoli	Green Onions	Fennel
Brussel sprouts	Kale	Lettuce
Cabbage	Kohlrabi	Olives
Cauliflower	Mushroom	Radicchio
Chard	Rhubarb	Radishes
Chicory root	Sauerkraut	Romaine lettuce
Collard greens	Scallions	
Hearts of palm	Spaghetti squash	
Leeks	Spinach	
Lentils	Squash	
Okra	Tomato	
Onion	Turnips	
Peas	Zucchini	
Pea pods		
Peppers		
Pumpkin		
Water chestnuts		

Note: All of these vegetables provide a good source of fiber.

What Can We Eat Between Meals?

In our goal to lose weight, we want to restrict our caloric intake without feeling excessively deprived. In between lunch and dinner, therefore, there are some foods you may snack on.

But be aware that these foods occasionally slow down weight loss in some people and may need to be avoided in the first two weeks. If you seem to be losing weight slowly, you should moderate your intake of snacks.

Good Snack Foods

3 bread sticks
½ cup cereal
3 dates
3 graham crackers
5 pieces of melon (1 slice)
2 handfuls of peanuts (30-50)
10-20 almonds, cashews, or pistachios
2 cups air-popped popcorn
1 large pretzel
3 rice cakes
10 tortilla chips
half a small avocado
10 to 20 olives
an ounce of sour cream

Free Foods

Free foods are the so-called "sugar-free" or no-calorie foods.

Chewing gum (sugarless)

Herb tea (without barley or any fruit sugar added)

Lemon juice or lime juice (2.8 grams carbohydrate per ounce)

Clear broth/bouillon (read the label!)

Sugar-free gelatin

Regular water

Any of the following:

Decaffeinated coffee or tea

Club soda

Diet soda

Flavored seltzer

Sparkling water

Free Foods

Remember, you should eat no more than one snack during the day. There are, however, a few foods that have no calories and are called "free foods," which you may have as much of as you wish.

Getting Started: The First Few Weeks

Eat three meals and a snack every day. Don't skip meals! You'll get too hungry and may overeat.

Now that we know more about good and bad foods, the importance of restricting our caloric intake, and how many servings of each food group to eat each day, it is time to get started on our diet.

First, we need to increase our intake of protein and decrease our bad carbohydrate intake. For example, a good breakfast would include an egg and low-fat bacon or sausage. It is best not to eat bagels because they are high in carbohydrates and calories. Wheat toast is a good alternative. High fiber cereals are also a good choice. Look specifically for cereals with a low calorie content, high fiber content, and a good protein content. These options are a very good start to the day, particularly if eaten with skim milk, which increases the protein intake even further. An omelet with vegetables or bacon and ham is also a reasonable breakfast.

Dieting requires you to take careful inventory of what you eat but also when and how you eat. The guidelines in the box on this page provide a number of useful tips for planning your eating.

Keep in mind that you can approach losing weight in two ways:

1) For fast results, lose as much in the first two weeks as possible; or

2) Lose weight gradually.

The key is reducing the amount of food intake in the first weeks, so that the stomach does not dilate (or stretch) too much. The craving for excess food will stop.

Guidelines

1. Avoid bad carbohydrates. These include all white (bleached) flour carbohydrates, as well as white sugar carbohydrates.

2. Avoid saturated fats. Use olive or canola oil for cooking instead of butter or margarine. Introduce more polyunsaturated fat, like olive oil, into your meals. Olive oil helps decrease LDL, the bad cholesterol, and adds flavor to your food.

3. Introduce other types of ingredients for your salad dressing that have a low-fat and low-carbohydrate content, such as balsamic vinegar, which is very low in calories.

4. If you have an omelet in the morning or a hamburger at dinner, try not to use ketchup, mayonnaise, or other condiments high in carbohydrates. Use, instead, salsa because it contains vegetables and fiber and is low in carbohydrates and calories.

5. Gently grill your salmon, chicken, steak, or hamburgers, and try to use low-fat, lean meat.

Monitor Your Progress

To monitor your progress, please copy the sheet on the next page and record your food intake for the next three weeks. You need to write down every food that you eat and the amount you are consuming. You also need to write down what type of exercise you are doing and the length of time you are engaging in it. Please record your weight in the space provided but do not weigh yourself more than once a week. Also record any medications you are on and any problems you are experiencing; in this way, you have a record of your weight loss and the progress you are making toward your goal weight.

At the end of every week, analyze your progress chart. Did you eat the recommended servings per food group? Did you exercise regularly? Did you remember to drink lots of water.

Did you lose weight? If not, can you determine why? If necessary, calculate the calories per day that you consumed. Did you stay within your goal of 1500 or 1800 calories per day? Were there hidden calories that made you go over the recommended daily amount?

For the first three weeks, you need to write down every food that you eat and the amount you eat.

Weeks Three and Four

Continue following the suggested number of servings per day by food group from Chapter 11. After two weeks, you may be tempted to eat more. Please be careful, and do not overeat. Also, do not eat food the kids have left on the table just because you do not want to throw it away. Kids' foods, like chicken fingers, French fries, and pizza, can be detrimental to the concepts of the diet. Go to the supermarket and do your own food shopping, avoiding processed foods.

Weeks Five and Six

When your food cravings have stopped and you have completed the first few weeks of the diet, some foods can be reintroduced. For example, you will be able to eat more bread and good starches, like vegetables and fruit. It would also be good to start eating oatmeal and other cereals in the morning, particularly those with a high fiber content, but do not overdo it. Plan to eat good carbohydrates for one meal and only a small amount of carbohydrates with the other two meals.

Ideal Daily Meal Plan To Lose Weight

Below is an ideal meal plan, with a proper balance of protein, carbohydrates, and fat, to use in your diet:

Breakfast:

1. 6 ounces orange juice
2. 1 slice toasted wheat bread
3. 1 hard boiled egg or meat
4. No sweets.

Lunch:

1. Chicken sandwich with 2 ounces of meat (1 piece of bread and 2 pieces of meat)
2. Tomatoes or lettuce
3. 1 cup milk
4. ¼ cup cantaloupe.

Snack:

1. 2 cups of popcorn or 3 bread sticks
2. Diet soda.

Dinner:

1. 2 ounces boiled fish or meat
2. 1 small baked potato
3. Other vegetables, ½ cup of broccoli or ½ cup zucchini
4. 1 apple, pear, or other fruit
5. 1½ ounces of a dairy product
6. 5 to 6 whole-grain Saltine crackers

Later

You may have lost those 15-20 pounds that you needed to lose, and you may want to start eating again. Remember, your body is not going to see your weight loss as a positive event. If your body feels that the weight loss is a temporary stress, it will try to regain the weight. Therefore, you will not only regain the 15-20 pounds that you lost, you may gain an additional 20 or more pounds.

This is understandable because our bodies respond to an immediate weight loss with a stress response, which is to protect the body from the next food shortage or famine. However, if this happens, you have not only failed your diet, but you have also gained even more weight.

Sweets and Chocolate

After completing these steps, you can gradually reintroduce sweets, such as chocolate, into your diet. People love chocolate, and, in moderation, it is actually beneficial. Dark chocolate has been shown to have an effect on lowering cholesterol. Milk chocolate does not carry the same benefits and is more caloric, so if you crave chocolate, be sure to try eating dark chocolate. Do not eat a whole piece of chocolate, just a bite. A substitution for real chocolate is not as enjoyable or filling and can create other problems; therefore, eat real chocolate and do not feel guilty about it!

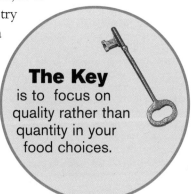

The Key is to focus on quality rather than quantity in your food choices.

	Morning Meal	Noon Meal	Evening Meal	Snacks	Activity	Weight	New Medicines	New Problems
Sunday								
Monday								
Tuesday								
Wednesday								
Thursday								
Friday								
Saturday								

Let's Start to Change Our Daily Habits

Shop smarter by sticking to the outer aisles of the supermarket. This is where you will find the fruits and vegetables, cheeses, meats and fish, cold cuts, breads, milk, dairy products, and fruit juices.

The best place to start changing the way we eat is not at the table or even in the kitchen, but at the supermarket. As I mentioned earlier in this book, it is easy to shop smarter simply by sticking to the outer aisles. This is where you will find the fruits and vegetables, cheeses, meats and fish, cold cuts, breads, milk and other dairy products, and fruit juices. If you can avoid the middle aisles with their sodas, snacks, and other highly processed foods, you will be halfway toward your goal of eating healthier food.

Shop Smart

When you open your refrigerator, it should be almost empty, with no sweets. If you want a snack, eat something else low in fat, such as vegetables or fruit, because that is what is in the refrigerator. If you ever watch any of the television programs that show the homes of fit people, you will notice that most of them have water and fruits and vegetables in their refrigerators. They do not have sodas, ice cream, snacks, and other types of unhealthy foods on their shelves. When there is stress, many people tend to eat whatever is in the house. If none of these temptations are in your house, you will not eat these foods. Fit people know that if they want to maintain their slim figures, they cannot have high calorie foods in the house.

If we bring home better food, we can rid ourselves of bad eating habits. We and our whole family will eat better, especially our children. Teenage and pediatric obesity are an increasingly severe problem in our society.

Fiber

A diet with plenty of whole grain products, vegetables, and fruit is optimal to our health. Fiber decreases the chance of constipation, diverticulitis, hemorrhoids, heart attacks, stroke, and some colon cancers. You can add a soluble fiber to your diet, such as vegetable juice, which is better than fruit juice because it contains less sugar and more fiber. Additionally, the skin on fruit is a good source of fiber, so it is important not to peel the skin off fruit.

A good source of fiber is one that provides at least two grams of fiber per serving. How much fiber do you need per day? Twenty to 35 grams of fiber, with a mix of both soluble and insoluble fiber, is a good goal. Soluble fiber-containing foods include vegetables, such as legumes. If you eat less fat, fewer carbohydrates, and increase your amount of exercise and fiber intake, you will definitely lose weight. On the other hand, if you eat more fat, more calories, and exercise less, you will gain weight.

Buy Smaller Clothes

Another simple strategy for losing weight is to get rid of your larger clothes and buy clothes that are smaller than you are. It is important, however, not to be unrealistic in your clothing purchases. Don't buy a size 6 dress when you wear a size 14; instead, buy a size 12 dress, and when you are able to wear that size comfortably, purchase a size 10 dress, and so on. The new clothes will feel a bit tight, and you will feel that you have to lose more weight. On the other hand, if you keep the larger clothes, you will feel that you have enough room to indulge in certain foods. So clean out your closet. Donate your larger clothes to women's shelters or other charities and buy new clothes that are tighter and that are more in line with your desired body image.

People who eat alone tend to eat more.

Eat With Your Family

Another strategy that will enhance your family life as well as help keep your weight in check is to have as many family members as possible present at mealtime. The social interaction will make eating an enjoyable, relaxing experience, where conversation will become more of a focus than the amount of food consumed.

My Mom's Principles

When I was visiting Italy, my mother provided me with some additional suggestions for eating wisely. Although she is not a physician, she has tremendous common sense and an excellent understanding of the needs of the human body. Typically, she eats four small meals a day and is very careful not to overindulge in food. She is in excellent shape and health.

- Drink water all day long.
- Eat slowly and chew properly.
- Always leave the table slightly hungry. Don't stuff yourself.
- Do not mix too many foods because this will make your digestion difficult and unsatisfying.

Stop Sugar Cravings

Americans consume 10 million tons of sugar annually and account for 33 percent of the world's sugar consumption, even though they make up just 5 percent of the world's population. In France, a country known for its delectable pastries, the yearly sugar consumption is 88 pounds per person compared to 158 pounds consumed per person in the U.S. Clearly, Americans eat far too much sugar, and this contributes to our problems with obesity.

The Keys
to Moderating Sugar Intake

1. Fill up the stomach, so that there will be less of an urge to overeat.

2. Eat something to decrease the acidity in the stomach, such as fat or fiber.

How can we stop our craving for sugar? Reviewing the following points made in Chapter 8 on foods that make us feel full and foods that make us feel hungry will assist us.

Sweets, fried foods and acidic foods make us feel hungry.

To feel full:

1. Fill up and distend the stomach, so that there will be less of an urge to overeat because the stomach is full.

2. Eat something to decrease the acidity in the stomach and prevent insulin levels from rising too quickly such as fiber or fat in moderation. Thus, follow these suggestions:

Increase the distention of the stomach before eating.

Increase fiber intake.

Increase fat intake in moderation.

Fill Up the Stomach

My mother, a wise and fit woman, recommends drinking one or two glasses of water before each meal. This distends the stomach and gives it a feeling of fullness. When your meal is served, your craving for food, including those items loaded with sugar, will be diminished. When filling up a stomach already distended with water, there will be less of an urge to overeat because the stomach is already full and is not acidic.

Soda Versus Water Principles

You need to understand the difference between carbonated drinks and water. When you drink sodas, because of the gas and acidity, the stomach will be distended because of the gas, but the acidity is also increased. If acidity increases, there is a higher possibility to become hungrier because acid increases the requirement of food. However, if you drink water, the water is not acidic and the water will not stand on your stomach. The stomach does not feel the acidity— it feels full, yet hunger is not increased.

Increase Fiber Intake

Fiber is good because, like fat, it takes longer for the stomach to process this substance and for the intestine to digest it. Thus, we feel full for a longer period of time. At the same time, we do not increase our insulin too much because the content of sugar found in fiber is not excessive. My mother, for example, suggests eating a big serving of green salad before a meal because it will fill up the stomach. The application of dressing should be minimal because dressing can increase your appetite.

Use Fat to Diminish Hunger

The acid in the stomach, in part, makes us hungry; we neutralize this acid by eating. Fat in moderation is especially good at neutralizing acidity and diminishing hunger. The fat also has a slow progression through the intestine; therefore it takes longer to digest it, and you feel full for a longer period of time.

Fruit Alone Increases Hunger

People often eat fruit peeled before their meal because they think it will make them feel full. However, this is not the case because fruit has sugar, and the more sugar that is ingested, the more the insulin levels rise. And the more insulin levels go up, the more sugar the stomach requires. The sugar in fruit is easy for the stomach to digest and does not leave the stomach distended; therefore, more food is needed to satisfy your hunger cravings.

Fruit juices are even worse since they contain a lot of sugar. They are absorbed very quickly, which means insulin is going to go up very quickly, while the acidity remains in the stomach. Not only does the gastric acid stay in the stomach, requiring more food to neutralize it, but most juices are acidic. As a result, the acidity in the stomach actually increases, and the stomach will need even more food to compensate for it.

What About Coffee?

Coffee has two opposite actions: The warm temperature will dilate the stomach and at the same time, the caffeine is acidic, thereby increasing the acidity and hunger.

A moderate amount of coffee provokes temporary changes in the cells of the gastric mucous and dampens the desire for food. If we put a lot of milk in coffee, however, we decrease the appetite-suppressing effect of the coffee. A large amount of milk makes the coffee move more slowly to the small intestine, so it sits longer in the stomach and induces further acidity.

Action of Surgery

Similar results occur after surgery to treat morbid obesity. The surgery is performed in two ways:

1. Restricting the stomach to decrease its size; and

2. Bypassing part of the intestine to decrease the intake of calories.

The restriction of the stomach makes the patient feel full quickly, so he or she does not have the desire to continue eating. If you have a gastric bypass only some parts of the intestine are bypassed; if too much is bypassed, serious side effects, including liver disease, result.

Eating Out

Get salad dressing on the side and dip the fork, not the food, into the dressing.

Although some restaurants are beginning to serve healthier food, eating out poses a real challenge when it comes to staying on a diet or even simply maintaining an optimum weight. Here are some great tips to remember when dining out.

Portion Sizes

Portion sizes at restaurants are often enormous, so be sure to take note of the portion sizes people are eating as you walk into the restaurant. If they look big, ask for a child's or a half portion when ordering. Consider splitting an entrée with your dining partner.

Salads

Without realizing it, we tend to consume a lot of our calories during meals from our salad dressings. There are many types of dressings: Blue Cheese, French, Thousand Island, and Ranch, to name a few, but they are all high in calories. Moreover, many people add cheese, peanuts, bacon bits, and bread croutons to their salads, which contribute even more calories.

You should avoid these add-ons and order your dressing on the side. When applying the dressing, limit yourself to just a few dots of dressing here and there. Do not empty the entire cup of dressing that you were given. You will find that the salad tastes the same because you taste the dressing right away. Dip your fork in the dressing, and

Tips for Dining Out

1. Check out restaurants prior to eating out and have a list of appropriate places that meet your needs.
2. When possible, select restaurants offering low-fat items.
3. Eat slowly. Pick restaurants that allow you time to dine, not eat and run.
4. Order a child's plate or a "lite" plate or split an entrée with your dining partner.
5. Ask for a "to go box" when you order your meal. Divide the food in half at the start of the meal, and take the rest home for the next day.
6. Select plain, broiled, or baked items.
7. Ask your server how the food is prepared.
8. Ask for sauces, gravies, condiments, or dressing to be left off your plate or put them on the side.

then eat the salad. Or better yet ask for a little bit of olive oil and balsamic vinegar–these are a healthier addition than most salad dressings. This is an easy and painless way to cut an amazing two-thirds of the calories from your salad!

Appetizers

Try to get regular-sized instead of double-sized appetizers or, better yet, avoid them altogether.

Beverages

If you are drinking wine, be sure to order it by the glass rather than by the bottle, because you can pace yourself better. If you buy it by the bottle, you may have a tendency to drink more, therefore, consuming more calories. Alternate alcoholic beverages with non-alcoholic ones, such as club soda or water. Dilute your drink with club soda, as in a wine spritzer, to give yourself more volume and less alcohol. Ask for liquids without ice or ice separately. You can better measure the amount of liquid if there is no ice.

Below are some of the foods to stay clear of at various types of restaurants:

Foods to Avoid

There are also a lot of foods that should be completely avoided when eating out. Fat is abundant in foods like fettuccini Alfredo and anything that is butter-dipped, breaded, creamy, deep fried, marinated, sautéed, or "braised in its own juices." Avoid combo foods, super, grandé, king-size, and supreme.

Chinese Food

Buttery foods, fried foods, crispy foods, noodles, sweet and sour dishes, sweet duck sauces, and twice-cooked dishes are especially caloric. Fish, shrimp, scallops, and all spices are fine. Twice cooked dishes are especially bad because they have a lot of calories.

Deli Foods

At the deli, eat less bologna, corned beef, eggplant or chicken Parmesan, extra cheese, pastrami, meatballs, and salami. Eat more ham, carrots, raisins, mustard, pickles, chicken, and tuna. Try not to eat cheese sauce or chicken nuggets, which are processed and bleached dark meat, and which often include the skin. Avoid crescent sandwiches, fried chicken or fish, jumbo-sized fries, and onion rings.

Diners

Eat grilled chicken, fat-free or low-fat salad dressing, a single burger, and a regular side of kids' fries or small fries. Instead of eating baked potatoes, eat sweet potatoes because they contain fewer calories than baked potatoes. Diners usually serve both. Avoid the butter and sour cream that are so often used as toppings on baked potatoes.

French Food

Among the foods to avoid at French restaurants are the French au le crème, au gratin, and mayonnaise-based foods. Good foods are steamed, boiled, or grilled.

Indian Food

Indian restaurants are good if you eat curried food, peas, and rice. Avoid eating anything that is made with butter, such as ghee, korma sauce, or molee sauce, which is found in coconuts. Deep-fried bread or samosas, which are a fried appetizer, are very high in fat.

Italian Food

In Italian restaurants, do not eat dishes with Alfredo sauce because there is too much cream and butter. Also avoid fried eggplant and zucchini. Pasta is very good with light red sauce, marinara sauce, or ricotta cheese. When ordering pizza, avoid extra cheese, meatballs, pepperoni, and sausage toppings. Most importantly, watch the portion sizes of all food served.

Japanese Food

In Japanese restaurants, stay away from agemono, deep-fried katsu, fried pork cutlet, and sukiyaki, a meal containing beef fat, and tempura, which is fried. Anything steamed is good (mushimono, nabamo, nimono, sashimi, sushi, yaki fu), as is anything grilled.

Mexican Food

Healthy Mexican food choices include black bean soup, scallops, fish, chili and fajitas. Avoid refried beans, chimichangas, and tortilla shells.

Thai Food

When eating Thai food, stay away from foods containing coconut, peanuts, and metrob (crisp dinner rolls), which are all high in fat and calories.

Let's Talk About Exercise

We should never lose sight of the fact that exercise is a major component of weight loss because it keeps us healthy and lowers our cravings for food. When you exercise, you become tired and this decreases your appetite, thereby restricting your food intake. The hips and waist are the first places you may lose weight, and you will start feeling good about this because your waistline decreases one or two sizes.

> You need to exercise at least three times a week, and your activity needs to last 20 to 30 minutes.

Exercise is also a good means of avoiding a whole host of potential health problems. The major complications of being overweight are diabetes, heart problems, and atherosclerosis. We have already discussed bad and good cholesterol. If you have high bad cholesterol (LDL), low good cholesterol (HDL), high blood pressure, obesity, and high triglycerides, you are at the highest risk of having a heart attack and atherosclerosis. You should be thoroughly checked by your doctor before embarking on any exercise program.

High Intensity

In order for exercise to confer its maximum benefits, the intensity of the exercise must be high. Walking without focusing on the walk will not make you lose weight; you must walk briskly, not meander. The only way to lose weight is to increase your heart rate by at least an additional one half or three quarters of normal. If your heart rate is 70 beats per minute, you should obtain a heart rate of 110 to 120 when you exercise (a 40% to 50% increase). When you exercise and increase your heart rate, your metabolism increases; thus, more sugar and energy are burned.

Sweating Is a Good Thing

Why do some people sweat more than others? If you sweat, it means that your heart rate is up. If your heart rate is up, your metabolic rate is up, and if your metabolic rate is up, you are losing weight. Everyone exercises differently; there is no magic time or number. However, you do need to exercise at least three times a week, and your activity needs to last 20 to 30 minutes.

What Exercise Is Best?

The best exercise is an activity you enjoy doing; you will be much more likely to stick with it day after day, year after year. Walking is one of the easiest exercises to engage in because it can be done anywhere—your neighborhood, a park, on city sidewalks—and it requires no special equipment other than a good pair of shoes.

Start Slowly and Build

To avoid injury when first starting out, you should begin slowly and gradually increase the intensity and length of your exercise activity. Again, remember that you should not start an exercise routine without seeing a physician first.

The best exercise is an activity you enjoy doing; you will be much more likely to stick with it day after day, year after year.

The list below illustrates various activities and the calories burned in 20 minutes of engaging continuously in that activity.

20 Minutes of Exercise	Calories
Football	220
Scrubbing the floor	180
Aerobic dance	130
Ballroom dancing	84
Cleaning	102
Pushing the mower	186
Walking	134
Running 9 minutes/mile	320
Squats	252
Jumping rope and running	72
Basketball	220
Cross country skiing	198
Raking	90
Mopping the floor	102
Rock climbing	249
Racquetball	296
Tennis	180

According to an old Roman saying "mens sana in corpore sano," meaning healthy mind in healthy body.

An example of the Exercise Flow Chart used at our weight loss clinic has been provided for you in Appendix 2 to help give you an idea of how to evaluate your readiness for physical activity and to help you keep track of your progress.

Do What the Italians Do

I am confident that the philosophy and lifestyle suggestions learned from this book will help you to lose weight, but more important to keep the weight off and stay slim, by modifying your behavior and by understanding that food is a friend and not a foe. The modified Italian diet will provide you with the right amounts of protein, fat, and carbohydrates. This diet tastes good and moderates food intake, but does not restrict the types of food eaten. You can eat well and enjoy eating while losing weight. It is important when you start the diet to remain disciplined about portion size and the amounts of fat and carbohydrates you consume.

Do what the Italians do—eat good food but not too much.

If you do not stop the vicious cycle of your body needing food, you will never rid yourself of the urge that keeps pushing you to eat more. We all know that it is important to identify and all but eliminate the bad carbohydrates found in refined white breads, highly processed cereals, cakes and cookies. However, even the fiber-rich, good carbohydrates are still turned into glucose by our bodies, so be careful not to overindulge in fruits or vegetables that contain a high percentage of carbohydrates, such as grapes and corn.

The key is to permanently change your eating habits, particularly in regard to portion sizes and the amount of calories, carbohydrates, and fats you eat. These changes will not only keep you slim, but they will also make you healthy. And being healthy is absolutely priceless; there is no greater reward.

In your approach to food, just "do what the Italians do." Eat good food but not too much. Do not double the size of your portions. Modest servings of pasta are fine as long as they are topped with healthy tomato sauce, fish, or vegetables, not the fattening sauces found in so many restaurants. Olive oil and good carbohydrates, like those contained in green vegetables and salad, are excellent to eat. It is also a good idea to eat different types of foods that help reduce the acidity of the stomach and slow digestion, like green beans and fava beans. If fiber is absorbed slowly, the insulin levels will not increase rapidly, and this will decrease the need for more food.

From: Mitch, Texas

I applied Dr. Frezza's diet. In the first week, I lost 8 pounds and in 30 days, I lost 20 pounds. What shocked me about his diet are the simple ingredients that have been used and the fact that fresh ingredients can make a difference, making your food tastier. Therefore, you use less salt, butter or ingredients that are fattening or that can have an impact on weight increase. I would recommend this diet to anyone who needs to lose 20-30 pounds.

The Key is to permanently change your eating habits, particularly in regard to portion sizes and the amount of calories, carbohydrates and fats you eat.

For dessert, avoid extremely sweet food. What about ice cream? You can eat two to four teaspoons of ice cream with fresh fruit or you can eat a little more of a low-fat, low-carb ice cream.

If you eat fast food, eat chicken and avoid high calorie condiments such as mayonnaise or ketchup. Also drink water or coffee. Stay away from the high-sugar sodas.

Much of this diet is based on common sense. Moderation in portions and calories are fundamental not only in helping you to lose weight, but also in maintaining your optimum weight. And when you moderate your intake through the techniques you have learned here, you can eat good food and enjoy every bite without feeling guilty or deprived.

From: Kari, Texas

I had problems with weight gain, but I could not undergo bariatric surgery. Dr. Frezza was kind enough to take me as a patient and suggested several options for me. His diet was a revelation. I never believed that my weight problem was secondary to the fact that I was misbehaving towards the food. I was eating my kid's leftovers; therefore, I was not controlling my eating habits. After trying his diet and philosophy, I understood that modifying my habits during the day was enough to control my food intake. This helped me in the first 5 weeks to lose 21 pounds. I would recommend his diet to anyone.

From: Jennifer, New Mexico

I was gaining weight because I was overcooking my food. I liked the taste of the food and I could not eat food that did not taste good. When I talked to Dr. Frezza about gaining weight, I realized a simple way to solve this problem was using different ingredients, eating fresh foods instead of processed foods. His second suggestion worked as well, which was to buy new clothes. I bought smaller-sized clothes and because they were a little too tight, I worked very hard to lose more weight following his diet suggestions. I applied his formula and it worked. I was able to lose 19 pounds in 6 weeks.

Eating well is the key to healthy living, or as the Italians say "vivere sani mangiando bene" —live well by eating well.

Recipes
"From our family to you"

PLEASE TAKE NOTICE

Recipes are made to be good!

Ingredients can be exchanged

but at times a little bit of an original recipe is

better than a lot of a modified one!

Enjoy, but control yourself.

ANTIPASTI

The word antipasto means "before the meal" and traditionally consists of a selection of fresh and quickly prepared foods. All of the dishes featured in this section are also perfect as a light meal, supper or brunch.

A delicious and very simple creation by Giuseppe Cipriani, founder of Harry's Bar in my home city of Venice. The version featured here uses steak and Porcini mushrooms but you can also experiment with veal, tuna or swordfish and arugula (instead of mushrooms).

Carpaccio

1 lb. very fresh filet of steak*
1 large lemon
8 small Porcini mushrooms (or small Champignons if you can't find Porcini)
3 oz. shavings Parmigiano Reggiano cheese
3 or 4 tablespoons extra-virgin olive oil
salt and freshly-ground black pepper
1 tablespoon chopped flat-leafed parsley

* Ask your butcher to filet the steak into very thin pieces, as if it was ham, and against the grain of the meat. Raw steak is safe to eat as long as it is very fresh. Make and serve carpaccio on the same day. If you are experimenting with one of the fish alternatives, do not buy fish that has been frozen.

1. Arrange the filets on a large serving dish, with little overlap.
2. Make a dressing with the juice of 1 large lemon, the olive oil, salt and pepper. Sprinkle over the steak. Allow the juices to soak into the meat for about 15 or 20 minutes.
3. Slice the mushrooms thin and arrange them on top of the meat with some slices of Parmesan cheese. Sprinkle with chopped parsley.

Serves 4

Frittata (also as entrée)

4 eggs
2 zucchini, sliced thin
½ small onion
2 tablespoons extra-virgin olive oil
salt and freshly-ground black pepper
½ tablespoon fresh flat-leaf parsley, chopped

1. Heat 1 tablespoon oil in a skillet and sauté the zucchini slices and onion until they start to brown. Empty the vegetables into a bowl.
2. Beat the eggs and add them to the bowl. Add the salt, pepper and parsley. Mix thoroughly.
3. Add the second tablespoon oil to the skillet and as soon as it is heated, add the egg mixture. Turn the heat to low. Cook the eggs until they are almost set in the middle.
4. Flip the frittata upside down to cook on the other side or run the skillet under the broiler for a minute or so until the frittata has completely set. If you use a broiler, make sure that the handle on your skillet is flameproof.
5. Cut into small wedges and serve.

Serves 2

Frittatas are different than omelettes in that they are flatter, less creamy and never runny. In addition to a hearty appetizer, they also make for a great lunch or dinner when served with a simple green salad. This version is made with zucchini, but you can also experiment with any of the following: cheese, fresh basil cut into very thin strips, artichokes, mushrooms, potatoes, onions, sun–dried tomatoes, leftover pasta, spinach or zucchini flowers (one my family's favorite). Most frittatas are best served slightly warm. This particular version is also delicious cold.

Nonna Maria's Eggplant and Pepper Medley

This popular dish can be found on the antipasto tables of just about every region in Italy. The flavors and colors of peppers and eggplants mix very well together and make for a very appetizing presentation. As a variation on this dish, substitute roasted plum tomatoes for the eggplants. My wife's grandmother introduced me to this combination when I first visited her in Calabria . She always roasted the tomatoes on an open fire pit but a grill will work fine too.

2 long eggplants (Aubergines)
1 yellow pepper
1 red pepper
2 tablespoons extra-virgin olive oil
2 garlic cloves
½ teaspoon dried oregano
4 or 5 fresh basil leaves
4 teaspoons balsamic vinegar
salt and freshly-ground pepper

1. Slice the eggplants into slices about ¼ inch thick, sprinkle them with salt on both sides and leave in dish for 1 hour or more until they sweat all their bitter juice away. Then, wash the eggplants in running water and dry them lightly.
2. Roast the eggplants and the whole peppers on a grill or on a cookie sheet under a broiler flame. Cook until the skin of the peppers looks charred and blistered. The eggplants should soften and start to brown.
3. To remove the skin on the peppers more easily, put them in a paper bag and seal for about 30 minutes or so. The steam in the bag should loosen the skin. Peel or scrape off the skin. Then remove the core with the ribs and seeds inside the peppers. Slice into lengthwise strips about ½ inch wide.
4. Cut the eggplants also into strips about ½ inch wide and arrange them on a serving plate alternating them with the peppers. Sprinkle with salt and pepper.
5. Add oregano, crushed garlic cloves, olive oil and chopped basil leaves.

Serves 4

Prosciutto with Melon or Figs

8 slices paper-thin prosciutto
8 slices honeydew or cantaloupe melon

Wrap each piece of melon with a slice of prosciutto and serve.

8 slices paper-thin prosciutto
4 ripe, soft figs cut into halves
8 fresh mint leaves

1. Place mint leaf over fig half
2. Wrap each fig and mint leaf with prosciutto slice and serve.

Either version can be made several hours in advance and stored in the refrigerator until ready to serve. Serve at room temperature.

Serves 2 to 4

Prosciutto is an unsmoked, air-cured and salted ham made from the hind shank of a hog. It is very high in protein and has a slightly sweet, savory taste. If possible, look for prosciutto from the Parma region of Italy (known to be the best!). You'll recognize it by the crown symbol that is branded on each ham by the Consortium of Prosciutto di Parma as a guarantee of its quality. The pairing of prosciutto with melon is a very popular antipasto in Italy. Try it also with fresh figs.

Caprese Salad

Mozzarella cheese and tomatoes is a very popular summer dish in Italy. Use the best summer tomatoes you can find—preferably locally grown—and mozzarella made from the milk of a water buffalo if you can find it. With a slice or two of crusty bread it can also make a perfect lunch dish.

4 tomatoes
2 cups mozzarella cheese
fresh basil leaves
2 tablespoons extra-virgin olive oil
salt and freshly-ground black pepper

1. Slice the tomatoes and mozzarella into thick rounds. Arrange in overlapping slices on a dish, alternating between the cheese and the tomatoes.
2. Top with few basil leaves. Sprinkle with olive oil, salt and black pepper.

Serves 2 to 4

Sirenetta Seafood Salad

½ lb. shrimp with shell and dark vein removed
½ lb. cleaned squid
½ lb. fresh small clams
1 lb. fresh mussels
1 fennel bulb (remove the green top from the bulb) or 1
    stalk of celery
¼ cup extra-virgin olive oil
1 lemon
1 or 2 cloves garlic
½ cup dry white wine
2 tablespoons chopped flat-leaf parsley
1 bay leaf
salt and freshly-ground pepper

For this dish, use whatever is in season or a combination of fresh and frozen fish. For a heartier salad, you can add ¼ pound small red potatoes (boiled in salted water, peeled and cooled before cutting them into small pieces) and a sweet roasted pepper (cut into strips).

1. Bring a pot of water with 1 bay leaf to a boil. Add the shrimp and cook for about 2 minutes until they start to turn pink. Drain well and devain.
2. Drop the squid in the same water and cook for about 10 minutes until tender. Remove and allow to cool. Slice the main body of the squid into rings about ¼ inch wide. You can leave the tentacle section intact or slice into 2 pieces, if large.
3. Scrub and rinse the clams and mussels in cold water then place in a separate, covered sauce pan with the wine. Steam until all the shells have opened and lift the clams and mussels from the shells. Make sure you discard any shells that do not open. Do not try to force them open.
4. Place the shrimp, squid, clams and mussels in a large bowl. Cut the fennel or celery into small pieces and add them to the mixture.
5. Make a dressing using the oil, juice of 1 lemon, finely-chopped garlic, parsley, salt and pepper. Pour over the fish and fennel or celery and mix well. Serve slightly chilled.

Serves 6 to 8

SOUPS

This delicious soup is easy to make and makes the most of summer vegetables.

Italians can't get enough of zuppe, minestre, minestrine and minestrone! These can be a delicate starter course or a hearty and filling main meal. Invest in a good repertoire of Italian soups in your everyday cooking. It is one of the easiest ways to create a nutritious and complete meal. In this section, you'll find a few of my family's favorites.

Minestra Di Zucchini

3 tablespoons extra-virgin olive oil
1 lb. green zucchini and yellow squash
1 large onion, chopped
½ lb. tomatoes, diced
4 cups low-fat chicken stock or water
2 potatoes
2 tablespoons fresh flat-leaf parsley
salt and freshly-ground pepper
Optional: ½ cup freshly grated Parmigiano Reggiano
     cheese

1   Heat the oil in a large pot. Add the chopped onion and cook until soft. Add the tomatoes.
2   Chop the zucchini, squash and potatoes into coarse pieces. Stir into the pot with the onion and tomatoes. Allow to brown slightly.
3   Cover with the chicken stock or water and cook, bring to a boil and lower the heat to a simmer. Cook for 20 minutes or until the vegetables are tender. Stir frequently to prevent the vegetables from sticking to the bottom of the pot.
4   Garnish with fresh parsley and Parmgiano Reggiano cheese if desired.

Serves 4 to 6

My Family's Lentil Soup

2 cups dried lentils
1/3 cup extra-virgin olive oil
1 onion, finely chopped
2 garlic cloves
2 tablespoons chopped flat-leaf parsley
4 tablespoons tomato paste
1 stalk celery, finely chopped
1 slice pancetta, thinly sliced
4 salted anchovies, boned and chopped into small pieces
freshly grated Parmigiano Reggiano cheese for the table
salt and freshly-ground pepper
Optional: rind from a small piece of Parmigiano Reggiano cheese

Lentils are a good source of protein and highly nutritious. Look for an Italian variety called Castelluccio (from an area by the same name in Southern Italy). They are well worth the hunt!

1. Wash the lentils and let them soak in some warm water for 1 hour or so. Discard any lentils that float to the top. Drain the others and put them in a pot with 2 quarts of lightly salted water to cook. Add also the Parmigiano Reggiano rind if using. Bring to a boil and then reduce the heat to a simmer until the lentils are tender. Remember to stir the lentils from time to time to prevent sticking.
2. In a separate large pot, heat oil and add the onions and garlic. Cook for 2 or 3 minutes until they start to soften. Add the pancetta and the anchovies. When the pancetta and anchovies start to brown, add the tomato paste. Season with salt and pepper. If the mixture is too thick, dilute it with a spoonful or two of water. Simmer for 10 or 15 minutes.
3. While the savory base is simmering, puree half of the lentils in some of the liquid and return to the pot.
4. Pour the pureed lentils into the pot with the savory base.
5. Drain the lentils that you did not puree and add them to the savory base pot as well. Reserve the cooking water from the lentils. You will need it to soften the soup if it starts getting too thick. Adjust the seasoning if necessary and cook for an additional 10 minutes.
6. Ladle into individual soup plates and sprinkle with freshly-grated Parmigiano Reggiano cheese.

Serves 4 to 6

Venetian Bean Soup

Venetians often add a small pasta variety called ditalini in the last 10 minutes of step 3 and cook it with the soup until al dente. I, on the other hand, prefer to omit the pasta to cut down on calories. This rustic dish is very hearty and filling even without the pasta.

2 cups dried beans such as cannellini or cranberry beans
5 tablespoons extra-virgin olive oil
1 medium onion, chopped into small pieces
1 leek, sliced into thin pieces
1 thick slice smoked pancetta
1 small carrot, sliced
1 celery stalk, chopped into small pieces
½ cup canned Italian plum tomatoes
1 lb. swiss chard, cut into small thin strips
4 cups vegetable stock
2 tablespoons fresh flat-leaf parsley
salt and freshly-ground pepper
freshly-ground Parmigiano Reggiano cheese for the table

1. Soak the dried beans overnight.
2. Put the olive oil, chopped onion and leek in a large soup pot. Cook until they become soft and slightly golden. Add the pancetta and cook until it starts to brown slightly. Add the carrot and celery and cook for 5 to 10 minutes, stirring occasionally. Add the plum tomatoes. Cook for 5 minutes; then add the swiss chard. Stir occasionally to prevent sticking and cook on low heat for a few more minutes.
3. Add the vegetable stock, a little at a time, until you reach a satisfactory consistency. Season to taste with salt and freshly-ground pepper.
4. Sprinkle with parsley and Parmigiano Reggiano cheese before serving.

Serves 4 to 6

Patrizia's Chicken Soup

4 chicken thighs with skin removed to eliminate some of
   the fat
2 carrots, chopped into large pieces
2 celery stalks, chopped into large pieces
1 large onion, chopped
½ cup green beans, chopped into bite-sized pieces
1 ripe tomato, quartered
2 tablespoons extra-virgin olive oil
2 tablespoons fresh flat-leaf parsley
salt and freshly-ground pepper
Optional: 2 large boiling potatoes, peeled, washed and cut
   into small dices,

1. Heat olive oil in a large pot. Add the onion. When the onion begins to soften, add the carrots, tomato and celery pieces. Cook for 3 to 5 minutes; then add the chicken thighs. Allow the chicken to brown a bit.
2. Cover the vegetables and the chicken pieces with plenty of water and add salt and pepper to taste. Bring to a boil. Reduce the heat to a low simmer and cook for 1 hour until the vegetables are thoroughly cooked and the chicken meat begins to fall off the bone.
3. Carefully remove the chicken pieces from the pot. Puree the vegetables and the broth.
4. Return the pureed soup to the pot and add the green beans. (If you choose to the add potatoes, add them at this point.) Cook for 5 to 10 minutes until the green beans (and potatoes) become tender.
5. In the meantime, return to the chicken pieces and remove the meat from the bones. Shred the meat using your fingers or a fork. Add the shredded meat to the pot and cook for 2 or 3 more minutes, stirring constantly.
6. Sprinkle with fresh parsley before serving. And for an extra zip, squeeze a little fresh lemon juice into the soup.

Serves 4 to 6

My wife Patrizia came up with this flavorful and delicate version for our children one night. They had resisted eating chicken soup in the past because they did not like soup with large pieces of vegetables and meat with bones. She solved the problem by simply changing the presentation of the soup. Try it!

PASTA and PIZZA

Use fresh plum tomatoes for this recipe if available. If you have to substitute canned tomatoes, look for varieties imported from Southern Italy, such as San Marzano.

Italians take their pasta very seriously and prefer combinations that are not fussy. Everyday pasta dishes are complemented with simple sauces and make the most of fresh ingredients. Keep portions reasonable and contained. Always cook pasta "al dente," leaving a slight "bite" to it and never, ever rinse it after you drain it.

Basic Tomato Sauce

4 tablespoons extra-virgin olive oil
1 small onion, finely chopped
1 clove garlic, finely chopped
1 lb. fresh plum tomatoes (You can substitute canned if
    fresh are not available.)
1 bay leaf
1 tablespoon tomato puree
4 leaves fresh basil
salt and freshly-ground black pepper

1. Heat the oil in a saucepan. Stir in the onion and until it becomes almost translucent.
2. Add the garlic, tomatoes, bay leaf and tomato puree. Season with salt and pepper. Cook for 3 or 4 minutes. Then add the basil leaves and cook for 30 to 45 minutes longer under low heat, stirring occasionally.
3. Pass the sauce through a food mill. Reheat if necessary and pour over your favorite pasta.

Aglio E Olio
Pasta with Garlic and Oil

6 tablespoons extra-virgin olive oil (use the best quality
   available)
2 cloves garlic
4 tablespoons chopped fresh flat-leaf parsley
salt and freshly-ground black pepper
Optional: red pepper flakes and grated Parmigiano
Reggiano cheese

1. In a large frying pan, heat the oil and gently sauté the
   garlic until it starts to become golden (but not brown).
2. Stir in the parsley and red pepper flakes if using.
3. Pour your favorite long pasta into the pan (when it is
   barely "al dente") with the oil and garlic. Cook together
   for 2 or 3 minutes. Stir well to make sure all parts of the
   pasta are coated.
4. Sprinkle with Parmigiano Reggiano cheese if using.

You can use any kind of pasta for this dish, but long varieties such as spaghetti, fettucine or bucatini work best.

Green Pesto

2 garlic cloves
3 cups fresh basil leaves
3 tablespoons pine nuts
1 oz. fresh flat-leaf parsley
½ cup extra-virgin olive oil
¼ cup mixed grated percorino and Parmigiano Reggiano
   cheese
salt and freshly-ground pepper

1. Crush the basil, parsley and garlic using a pestle and
   mortar or food processor. Process until you get a thick
   paste.
2. Add the cheese. Then proceed to add the oil in a thin
   drizzle.
3. Taste and adjust seasoning.
4. Spoon the pesto into the hot pasta and toss lightly.

Traditional Genoese pesto is made with pine nuts, but for an interesting variation try hazelnuts or walnuts instead.

Squid Pasta

After trying this dish, you'll probably agree with me that there's no better accompaniment to a fish-based sauce than artisanal pasta that is pre-infused with squid ink. The ink makes the pasta black in color and makes for a very elegant presentation. You can find it in any good Italian gourmet store.

1 tablespoon extra-virgin olive oil
2 tablespoons onion, finely-chopped
2 garlic cloves
1 lb. cleaned squid, cut into rings
½ cup dry white wine
8 chopped plum tomatoes with skin removed
1 lb. dried squid pasta such as tagliatelle or large penne
salt and freshly-ground black pepper

1. Heat the oil in a large skillet and add the onions and garlic. Cook until the onions start to become soft and the garlic a bit brown.
2. Add the squid. Stir and then cook for 3 or 4 minutes. Add the wine and simmer for an additional minute to give the wine an opportunity to evaporate.
3. Add the tomatoes, seasonings and most of the parsley. Cover and simmer for 45 minutes or until the squid is tender and a slightly dense sauce forms around them.
4. Cook the pasta until al dente. Drain and then add to the pan with the squid. Coat the pasta well with the sauce. Add the remaining fresh parsley and serve immediately while it is still hot.

Serves 6 to 8

Linguine Alla Carbonara

2 tablespoons olive oil
4 oz. pancetta or bacon, cut into very small pieces
1 tablespoon flat leaf parsley
5 or 6 egg yolks
2 tablespoons light cream
2 or 3 tablespoons freshly grated Parmigiano Reggiano
    cheese
salt and freshly-ground black pepper
1 lb. spaghetti

The ingredients in this luscious dish are not necessarily light and low in calories, so be sure to limit yourself to small portions. You can also omit the cream to cut calories further.

1. Heat the oil in a pan. Then add the pancetta or bacon and parsley. Brown the pancetta or bacon over medium heat.
2. In a bowl, beat together the egg yolks, cream and cheese.
3. Cook the linguine pasta al dente. Drain and turn it into the pan with the pancetta or bacon. Turn off the heat from under the pan.
4. Working quickly, add the egg and cheese mixture and toss to coat all the pasta with the sauce. The eggs will cook in the heat of the pasta.
5. Season with salt and pepper. Serve immediately while still hot.

Serves 6 to 8

Penne with Radicchio

Radicchio is a deep, red-leafed chicory. It has a slightly bitter taste and loses some of its color when cooked. Two varieties are available: one with elongated leaves from the city of Treviso and one with round-leafs from Chioggia. The latter is more readily available in the U.S. Combine it with pancetta or bacon, butter and cheese for an irresistible and delicious complement to pasta. You can also use it raw as a colorful and tasty complement to other ingredients in a fresh salad.

1 tablespoon extra-virgin olive oil
4 slices pancetta or bacon
3 heads of radicchio, shredded
1 tablespoon unsalted butter
2 tablespoons freshly grated Parmigiano Reggiano
1 lb. penne pasta

1. Cook the penne in a large pot of salted, boiling water.
2. While the pasta is cooking, sauté the bacon in a skillet over medium heat until it begins to brown. Add the radicchio. Cook for a few minutes until it begins to wilt. Add a couple tablespoons water if the radicchio starts to dry out.
3. Drain the pasta when it is al dente and transfer it to the skillet. Add the butter and cheese and toss to coat the pasta evenly.

Serves 6 to 8

Spaghetti with Tuna

1 6 oz. can Italian tuna, canned in olive oil
1 cup fresh tomatoes
1 clove garlic, finely chopped
4 to 6 black olives, pitted and chopped
½ teaspoon chili sauce
2 tablespoons flat-leaf parsley, finely chopped
½ lb. spaghetti
salt and freshly-ground pepper

A truly delicious pasta dish with simple ingredients.

1. Cook the spaghetti in a large pot of salted, boiling water until it is al dente
2. While the pasta is cooking mash the tuna with a fork in a large bowl. Add the tomatoes, garlic, olives, parsley, and chili sauce. Mix well and season to taste.
3. Reserve a few tablespoons the spaghetti's cooking water before draining.
4. Toss the spaghetti into the bowl with the tuna. Moisten the mixture with the reserved cooking liquid if necessary.

Serves 4

Fettucine with Salmon

In Italy, salmon is imported and quite expensive. While growing up, it was a dish reserved for special occasions. Here in the U.S., it is more readily available. It is also an excellent source of protein.

1 lb. green and white fettuccine
2 tablespoons extra-virgin olive oil
1 small onion, finely chopped
6 oz. Alaskan salmon cut into thin strips
½ cup light cream
½ cup dry white wine
5 tablespoons tomato puree
a pinch of freshly-ground nutmeg
2 tablespoons finely-chopped flat-leafed parsley
salt and freshly-ground pepper

1. Cook the fettuccine in a large pot of salted, boiling water until it is al dente.
2. While the pasta is cooking, heat the oil in a pan and cook the onion for 2 or 3 minutes. Then add the salmon in a pan and cook for another 6 minutes.
3. Add the white wine, tomato and continue to simmer over low heat. Slowly add the cream, nutmeg and parsley. Cook on low heat for a few minutes without letting the cream boil.
4. Drain the pasta and toss in the pan with the salmon and cream. Season to taste, mix well and serve.

Serves 6 to 8

Angel Hair Pasta with Vodka and Caviar

4 tablespoons olive oil
½ of a medium-sized leek
1 clove garlic, finely chopped
½ cup vodka
½ cup light cream
½ cup black caviar
1 lb. angel hair pasta
salt and freshly-ground pepper

Thin, angel-hair pasta is a perfect complement for this rather delicately-textured sauce. You may substitute spaghetti pasta if you prefer, but avoid rigatoni, penne and other short pasta that are better suited for heavier sauces.

1. Cook the angel hair pasta in a large pot of rapidly boiling, salted water until al dente.
2. Heat the oil in a frying pan. Add the leek and garlic and cook for 5 of 6 minutes.
3. Add the vodka and cream. Cook over low heat for a few more minutes.
4. Remove the pan from heat source and add the caviar.
5. Drain the pasta and toss with the caviar and vodka sauce. Adjust the seasoning if necessary.

Serves 6 to 8

Classic Pizza

The key to a great, Italian-style pizza is simplicity. Follow the advice of the Neapolitans whose pizza achievements are unequaled. Use fresh tomato sauce, the best mozzarella cheese you can find and tender basil. You'll find that delicious pizza is no further away than your own kitchen!

1 package dry yeast
1 cup + 2 tablespoons lukewarm water
a pinch of sugar
1 teaspoon salt
3 to 3 ½ cups unbleached white flour
fresh tomato sauce
2 tablespoons olive oil
salt and freshly-ground pepper
fresh mozzarella (preferably fior di latte mozzarella if you
     can find it)
fresh basil leaves cut into thin strips

1. Place the yeast in a medium-sized bowl. Add the 2 tablespoons lukewarm water and sugar. Mix well and allow to stand for a few minutes. The yeast will begin to foam.

2. Add all the salt and then flour a little at a time, waiting to incorporate the flour into the liquid before adding more. When the dough begins to form into a mass and pulls away from the sides of the bowl, remove it and place on a smooth work surface dusted lightly with flour. The dough should be dense and sticky. Add flour if it is too wet or water if it is too dry.

3. Knead the dough with your hands for about 20 minutes until it is soft and pliable. Form the dough into a ball.

4. Place the ball into a new, lightly-floured bowl. Cover with a clean kitchen cloth and allow to rise in a warm environment for 1 to 3 hours until the dough is doubled. If you do not have a wam place, you can warm your oven with medium heat for a few minutes, turn the oven off and place the bowl with the dough in the cooling oven. The dough will rise more easily in the oven.

5. When the dough has fully risen, return it to your work surface and punch it to release the air. Knead it for 5 minutes. Return it to the bowl and let it rise all over again for another hour or so.
6. After the dough has risen all over again, return it to your work surface. Cut it in half and roll each half into a thin circle about 10 to 12 inches in diameter using a rolling pin.
7. Place the dough onto a baker's peel if you are using a pizza stone. If you don't have a stone, you can use a slightly-oiled pizza pan or cookie sheet instead.
8. Cover the dough thinly but evenly with tomato sauce, then mozzarella cheese and fresh basil. Sprinkle with salt and pepper and drizzle the olive oil over the top.
9. Bake the two pizza for 15 minutes in a 500 or 550 degree oven until the crust is golden brown and the top is bubbling.

Serves 4 to 8

RISOTTO

Rice is eaten in many parts of the world, but risotto is unique to Italy. Its unique cooking method is what makes it distinctly Italian. This cooking method consists of a soffritto (sautéed base), the slow addition of broth and the use of rice varieties that grow only in Italy. The ingredients that flavor the rice can take many forms; everything from meat, vegetables, fish or even cheese. In Venice, the risotto tradition is especially strong and my family continues to make it quite often here in the U.S. Be sure to use Arborio, Carnaroli or Vialone Nano rice for your risotto recipes. If you try using long-grain rice, you will have a gooey mess.

Giovanni's Risi E Bisi

½ onion, finely chopped
1 rasher bacon fat
2 tablespoons parsley
1 tablespoon extra-virgin olive oil
2 tablespoons butter
½ lb. peas
5 cups chicken stock
2 cups Arborio, Carnaroli or Vialone Nano rice
½ cup grated Parmigiano Reggiano Cheese

1. Heat the oil and butter in a large pan and add the onion and bacon fat. Cook for 2 to 3 minutes until the onion starts to soften.
2. Add the peas and cook for an additional 5 to 7 minutes. Pour in all the stock and bring to a boil.
3. Add the rice and stir well. Cover and cook at a low simmer for about 15 minutes or until the rice takes on a creamy consistency. Stir frequently while the rice is cooking to prevent it from sticking to the bottom of the pot.
4. Remove from the heat and stir in the parsley.
5. Serve with grated Parmigiano Reggiano cheese on top.

Serves 4

Paolo's Risotto Alla Milanese

5 to 6 cups chicken stock
1 envelope saffron powder or 3 to 5 few saffron threads
5 tablespoons butter
1 small onion, finely chopped
1½ cups Arborio, Carnaroli or Vialone Nano rice
½ cup dry white wine
½ cup grated Parmigiano Reggiano cheese
salt

1. Bring the stock to a boil. Reduce to a slow simmer and put 2 or 3 tablespoons of this broth in a small bowl. Add the saffron and set aside to let it dissolve and infuse.
2. Melt 3 tablespoons butter in a large pot. Add the onion and cook until soft.
3. Add the rice and stir until all the grains have been coated with the butter and begin to swell. Add the wine and stir. Cook for a minute or two. Then add the stock a little at a time, waiting until the previous stock has been absorbed by the rice before adding more. Stir occasionally to prevent the rice from sticking to the bottom of the pot. The last stock added should be the stock with the saffron.
4. The risotto is ready when it is golden yellow, moist and very creamy, but not soupy. In Italy we call this consistency all'onda (meaning "like a wave"). When the risotto is ready, remove from the heat and add the remaining 2 tablespoons butter. Mix well. This last step will add to the voluptuous texture of the risotto.
5. Serve with Parmigiano Reggiano cheese grated on top.

Serves 4

This delicious risotto is a typical dish of Milan. It is flavored with saffron and makes for a delicious accompaniment to meat dishes such as pork roast or veal shanks (called osso buco in Italian). You can use canned chicken stock as indicated below or substitute home-made chicken stock made from chicken parts with bones, carrots, celery stalks, onions and ripe tomatoes for a more exquisite taste.

Risotto with Shrimp

12 oz. fresh shrimp in their shells
5 cups water
1 bay leaf
1 tablespoon chopped fresh parsley
1 teaspoon whole peppercorns
2 garlic cloves, finely chopped
5 tablespoons butter
2 shallots, finely chopped
1½ cups Arborio, Carnaroli or Vialone Nano rice
1 tablespoon tomato paste
½ cup dry white wine
salt and freshly-ground black pepper

Rice with fish is a Venetian tradition. The risotto can be done with any type of fish. Shrimp are easy to find in the U.S. and easy to cook. We chose this recipe to give a taste of a good risotto that is easy to make and very, very tasty.

1. Place the shimp in a large saucepan with the water, herbs, peppercorns and garlic. Bring to a boil and cook for 1 minute. Remove the shrimp, peel, and return the shells to the saucepan. Boil the shells for another 10 minutes. Strain. Return the broth to the saucepan and simmer until needed.
2. Slice the shrimp in half lengthwise, removing the dark vein along the back. Set 4 halves aside for garnishing. Roughly chop the rest.
3. Mix the tomato paste and wine.
4. Heat 3 tablespoons of butter in a frying pan. Add the shallots and cook until golden. Stir in the shrimp. Cook for 1 minute.
5. Add the rice, mixing well to coat it with the butter. After 1 to 2 minutes, pour in the tomato paste mixture. Raise the heat slightly and cook until the wine evaporates. Add the stock a little at a time, waiting until the previous stock has been absorbed by the rice before adding more. Stir occasionally to prevent the rice from sticking to the bottom of the pot. After about 20 minutes of cooking time, taste the rice. Season with salt and pepper as needed. Continue cooking, stirring and adding stock until the rice is al dente, tender but still firm to the bite. The total cooking time of the risotto may be from 20-35 minutes. If you run out of broth, use hot water. Do not worry if the rice is done before you have used up all the stock.
6. Remove from the heat and stir in 2 tablespoons butter. Garnish with the reserved shrimp halves.

Serves 4

Risotto Primavera

4 cups chicken stock
5 tablespoons butter
1 tablespoon extra-virgin olive oil
1 cup shelled fresh peas
1 cup fresh asparagus tips
2 small yellow squash, cut into small cubes
1 small onion, finely chopped
1½ cups Arborio, Carnaroli or Vialone Nano rice
½ cup grated Parmigiano Reggiano cheese
salt and freshly-ground black pepper

The colors in this risotto are a feast for the eyes. For variation use fava beans instead of peas and green beans instead of asparagus tips.

1. Melt the butter and the tablespoon of oil in a large pot. Add the squash and sauté for a few minutes until it begins to soften. Remove and set aside.
2. Add the onion and cook until soft.
3. Add the rice and stir until all the grains have been coated with the butter and begin to swell. Then add the stock a little at a time, waiting until the previous stock has been absorbed by the rice before adding more. Stir occasionally to prevent the rice from sticking to the bottom of the pot.
4. In a separate pot blanch the peas for 2 to 4 minutes. Drain and run under cold water to stop the cooking process. Drain again and set aside.
5. When the rice has finished cooking, stir in the remaining butter and then each of the vegetables.
6. Sprinkle each serving with grated Parmigiano Reggiano cheese.

Serves 4

Risotto with Strawberries

This is a very light yet luscious dish. The unusual combination of rice and strawberries makes a great conversation starter at dinner parties.

1 small onion, finely chopped
16 fresh ripe strawberries
3 tablespoons butter
2 cups Arborio, Carnaroli or Vialone Nano rice
½ cup dry white wine
2 cups vegetable stock
salt and freshly-ground pepper
2 tablespoons heavy cream

1. Melt the butter in a pot and add the onions. Cook until they start to soften. Then add all but 5 of the strawberries. Cook for a few more minutes until the strawberries begin to break down.
2. Add the rice to the pot and stir to coat all the rice. When the rice begins to puff add the white wine and cook for a minute longer. Then add the stock a little at a time, waiting until the previous stock has been absorbed by the rice before adding more. Stir occasionally to prevent the rice from sticking to the bottom of the pot.
3. Season with salt and pepper. When the rice is cooked, remove from the heat and add the heavy cream.
4. Serve with a garnish of fresh strawberry slices on top.

Serves 4

SALADS and VEGETABLES

Because so much Italian cooking is based on fresh ingredients, it is not surprising that there are lots of salads and vegetables in Italian kitchens and menus. Green salads make excellent accompaniments to main dishes. Whenever possible, do as the Italians do and buy vegetables only when they are in season. In other words, don't mix summer vegetables with winter vegetables in the same dish. This will be an easy way for you to keep your dishes varied and interesting throughout the year. You may also want to experiment with salads that include cooked vegetables, eggs or fish as a light meal all on their own. Raw vegetables provide excellent nutritional additions to daily diets providing Vitamin C and mineral salts.

This salad makes and excellent light meal with the added convenience that it can be quickly assembled from canned ingredients. If available, use imported tuna packed in extra-virgin olive oil. Drain the oil before adding to the salad mixture.

Tuna and Bean Salad

1 14-oz. can Cannellini beans, drained and rinsed under
    cold water
1 7-oz. can tuna fish, drained
2 tablespoons fresh lemon juice
2 tablespoons extra-virgin olive oil
1 tablespoon chopped fresh parsley or 1 teaspoon dry
    oregano
salt and freshly-ground black pepper

1. Place the beans and the tuna fish in a medium-sized mixing bowl.
2. In a separate small bowl make a dressing using the olive oil, lemon juice, salt and pepper and either the parsley or oregano. Mix well. Then add to the beans and tuna.
3. Toss well and serve.

Serves 4

Pinzimonio (Vegetable Dip)

Pinzimonio is typical dish from Rome. It features colorful assortment of vegetables served with a separate dish of extra-virgin olive oil, salt and pepper. You can also add a drop or two of balsamic vinegar in the dipping dish for an appetizing twist.

Assorted vegetables such as:
   carrots
   fennel bulbs
   green, red or yellow peppers
   celery
   scallions
   cauliflower or broccoli florets
   cherry tomatoes
   radishes
½ cup extra-virgin olive oil
2 tablespoons balsamic vinegar
salt and freshly-ground black pepper

1. Wash and cut the vegetables into matchsticks or bite-sized pieces.
2. Arrange the vegetables around a large platter, leaving room in the middle for a small dipping bowl.
3. In a small bowl mix the oil, vinegar, and salt and pepper. Place the bowl in the middle of the vegetable platter and serve.

Sautéed Peas with Onions

4 tablespoons finely-chopped onions
16 oz. shelled peas
2 or 3 tablespoons water
3 tablespoons extra-virgin olive oil
1 small cube vegetable buillon
salt and freshly-ground black pepper
Optional: pancetta or ham

1. Heat the oil in a medium skillet. If you are using pancetta or ham, sautè along with the onion for 3 or 4 minutes.
2. Stir in the fresh peas. Add water and buillon cube. Season with additional salt if necessary and a bit of freshly-ground pepper.
3. Cover and cook at medium heat until tender.

Serves 6

Use fresh peas (when in season) and onions to create this very tasty side dish to meat or frittate. You can also add a little ham or pancetta if you like.

Sautéed Zucchini

This is a very tasty dish cold or hot. You can use it as a sauce for pasta or omit the onions for a crispier and lightly-fried taste for the zucchini.

4 or 5 medium-sized zucchini
1 small onion, finely chopped
½ cup extra-virgin olive oil
2 tablespoons chopped fresh basil
1 tablespoon chopped fresh parsley
salt and freshly-ground black pepper

1. Cut the zucchini into thin ring-shaped slices.
2. Heat the oil in a skillet and add the onion. Sauté for a minute or two until soft, then add the zucchini.
3. Cook the zucchini until tender around the edges (probably 4 to 5 minutes).
4. Add basil and fresh parsley and cook for 1 minute longer.
5. Serve as a side dish or accompanied by a slice or two of fresh Italian bread.

Serves 4 to 6

Nancy's Summer Tomato Salad

6 large plum tomatoes
½ medium-sized red onion, finely chopped
3 or 4 tablespoons extra-virgin olive oil
finely-chopped basil or 2 teaspoons dried oregano
salt

1. Chop the plum tomatoes into small bite-sized pieces and put in a bowl.
2. Add the onion, basil or dried oregano. Salt to taste.
3. Drizzle olive oil over the mixture and toss well.
4. Allow the salad to sit at room temperature for ½ hour or so before serving so that flavors have a chance to absorb well.

Serves 4

This dish is often on the table at my mother-in-law's house during the summer. She uses fresh tomatoes from her garden and that makes all the difference. She usually alternates between fresh basil or dried oregano as a garnish. By adding some olives and tuna packed in olive oil (drained) you can quickly transform this salad into a wonderfully-colored and appetizing main dish.

Fennel, Tangerine and Arugula Salad

This light and refreshing salad combines both tart and sweet flavors as well as different textures.

2 tangerines separated into individual slices
1 fennel bulb
4 to 6 oz. arugula leaves
2 tablespoons extra-virgin olive oil
1 tablespoon balsamic vinegar
salt and freshly-ground black pepper
Optional: black olives

1. Cut the fennel bulb into very thin strips.
2. Combine in a bowl with the arugula leaves and tangerine slices.
3. Make a dressing using the oil, balsamic vinegar, salt and pepper. Pour over the salad and toss well. Add a few tasty black olives if you like.

Serves 4

Sauteed Eggplants with Garlic and Parsley

2 large eggplants, peeled and cut into ½ inch wide sticks
salt
1/3 cup extra-virgin olive oil
1 garlic clove, finely chopped
2 tablespoons chopped flat-leafed parsley

The key to a tasty eggplant is to first sprinkle the eggplant with salt and let it sit for 45 minutes or so to draw out the bitter juices.

1. Place the eggplant in a large bowl and sprinkle all pieces with salt. Cover with a dish or plastic wrap and add a weight to the top to exert light pressure on the eggplants. This will make it easier for them to release their bitter juices.
2. Drain the eggplants and pat dry on some paper towels.
3. Heat the oil in a large skillet at high heat. When the oil is hot, add the garlic and sauté slightly. Add the eggplants and cook until golden and soft (about 5 minutes or so).
4. Add the parsley and season with salt and pepper. Be careful not to add too much salt because some of the initial salt used to draw out the bitter juices may have lingered. Serve warm.

Serves 4

FISH

Baccalá (or salt-preserved codfish) is very versatile and economical. This particular recipe takes its name from the city of Vicenza. Because baccalá is preserved in salt, it requires soaking in several changes of water over a period of two days before it can be used. This process removes all excess salt from the fish and softens its flesh. You can also eliminate this step by purchasing pre-soaked baccalá from your fishmonger. Serve it with a couple pieces of crusty bread or alongside polenta.

Fish is very popular in Italy, especially in its many coastal towns. Opt for light and fresh sauces as well as recipes calling for quick cooking methods. Fish is rich in omega 3 acids. These are beneficial in controlling cholesterol and trygliceride levels. Fish is also an excellent source of protein. Find a good fish market and always evaluate a product's freshness before buying. The eyes should be bright and shiny. The flesh should be firm and slightly slimy. Open the gills and check to make sure that the flesh under these is still red or pink. Fresh fish will slightly smell fishy. A stale or strong fishy smell is a clear sign that the fish is not fresh.

Vicenza–Style Baccalá

2 lb. pre-soaked baccalá (cleaned and de-boned)
2 cloves garlic, very finely chopped
1/3 cup extra-virgin olive oil
1¼ cup 2 % milk
a pinch of grated nutmeg
salt and freshly-ground pepper

1. Place the fish in a deep skillet and cover it with cold water. Bring the water to a gentle boil and cook for about 5 minutes. Drain the water.
2. Sprinkle the baccalá with a few tablespoons olive oil and cook at medium heat, stirring frequently. The baccalà will begin to break into pieces. When it has fully absorbed all the oil, drizzle with a bit a milk and continue to stir until the milk is absorbed. Repeat these steps until all the oil and milk are gone. When finished cooking, the baccalà will look like a soft and light purée.
3. Season the fish with the grated nutmeg, salt, freshly-ground pepper and serve.

Serves 4

Rosa's Baccalá with Cherry Tomatoes

In this recipe, the baccalá is used as a salad and is best served at room temperature.

2 lb. pre-soaked baccalá, cleaned and de-boned
1/3 cup olive
1 lemon, sliced
3 cups cherry tomatoes, cut in half
2 tablespoons chopped fresh flat-leaf parsley
salt and freshly-ground pepper

1. Place the fish in a deep skillet. Cover it with cold water and add a couple thin slices lemon. Bring the water to a gentle boil and cook for about 10 to 15 minutes. Drain the water and allow the fish to cool to room temperature.
2. Remove the fish from the pan and cut into large cubes. Arrange the cubes on a deep platter along with the cherry tomatoes and parsley.
3. Whisk the oil with the salt, pepper and juice of the remaining lemon. Pour over the salad and serve.

Serves 4

Octopus with Lemon and Celery

When buying octopus, opt for small ones that are no more than 2½ lb. in weight. Anything bigger is likely to be tough in texture. The smaller the octopus, the more tender its meat. A Sicilian trick for tenderizing octopus while it is cooking is to add a cork from a wine bottle to the cooking water. The cork also helps to reduce the foamy scum that octopus usually produces while it boils. I don't have a scientific explanation for why this works, but it does. Try it!

2 lb. octopus (if buying whole ask your fishmonger to
     remove the eyes, beak and sacs)
2 tablespoons chopped fresh flat-leaf parsley
1 stalk celery, very finely chopped
4 tablespoons extra-virgin olive oil
4 tablespoons fresh lemon juice
salt and freshly-ground black pepper

1. Wash the octopus under cold running water and place it in a large sauce pan. Cover it generously with water and bring to a boil. Simmer for about 45 minutes until tender. Skim off any heavy foam that may rise to the surface.
2. Remove the octopus from the pan and allow to cool slightly. Slice the octopus into bite-sized pieces.
3. Place the octopus in a serving bowl and toss with the parsley, lemon juice, olive oil, celery and pepper. Mix well and allow to stand for a few minutes. Serve at room temperature.

Serves 6

Grilled Salmon with Fennel

4 medium salmon steaks
juice of 1 lemon
3 or 4 tablespoons the green fronds from the top of a fresh
    fennel bulb, chopped
4 tablespoons extra-virgin olive oil
½ teaspoon fennel seeds
salt and freshly-ground black pepper
4 lemon wedges

The mild flavor or cooked fennel goes very well with the strong flavor of salmon.
Be sure to remove any tiny pin bones from the salmon before cooking.

1. Put the salmon steaks in a bowl and coat them with a marinade made from the olive oil, lemon juice, fennel seeds and chopped fronds, salt and freshly-ground pepper.
2. Put the bowl in the refrigerator and allow to stand for 1½ to 2 hours.
3. Arrange the salmon steaks on a cookie sheet and broil each side for 4 to 5 minutes. When the edges of the salmon begin to brown, they are done.
4. Garnish with lemon wedges and serve.

Serves 4

Red Snapper "In Saor"

"In saor" is Venetian dialect for sweet-and-sour. The slightly sour taste of red vinegar mixed with the sweet taste of red onions and raisins are used in this recipe to create a seductive confiture for the red snapper. If you can't find fresh red snapper, you may substitute black sea bass or tuna.

2 large fillets red snapper (about 2 lb.)
6 tablespoons extra-virgin olive oil
1 very large red onion, thinly sliced
3 tablespoons red wine vinegar
1 teaspoon sugar
1 teaspoon pine nuts
1 teaspoon golden raisins
1 teaspoon freshly-grated orange zest

1. Heat 3 tablespoons olive oil in a large skillet. Sauté the onions until soft but not brown. Stir in the vinegar and cook for a couple minutes longer. Stir in the sugar, pine nuts, raisins and orange zest. Put aside until the red snapper is ready.
2. Brush the fillets with olive oil and place (skin side down) on a broiling pan or cookie sheet.
3. Broil the red snapper until lightly browned (5 to 7 minutes). Do not turn it.
4. Arrange the red snapper on a serving dish and spoon the onion confiture on top.

Serves 4 to 6

Tuna with Wild Mushrooms

¼ lb. wild mushrooms, chopped
4 small tuna steaks (about 1 to 1½ lb.)
2 tablespoons chopped fresh flat-leaf parsley
5 anchovy fillets
6 tablespoons olive oil
3 garlic cloves, minced
1 cup dry white wine
juice of ½ lemon
salt and freshly-ground black pepper

This is a very tasty dish, with strong flavors. Keep the portions small because tuna is a slightly fattier fish than most.

1. Heat the oil in a large pan. Add the mushrooms, anchovy fillets and garlic. When the anchovies have dissolved in the oil and the garlic starts to brown slightly, add the wine. Bring the mixture to a boil then lower to a simmer.
2. Add the tuna steaks and cook them for about 5 to 7 minutes, turning them over once.
3. Add the parlsey, salt, pepper and lemon juice and cook for a couple minutes longer.
4. Serve at once on a heated serving platter.

Serves 4

Livornese-Style Mullet

Mullet has a very savory, succulent taste and can be prepared in a number of ways including baking in parchment paper packages.

6 mullet, cleaned
3 tablespoons flour
4 tablespoons extra-virgin olive oil
2 crushed garlic cloves
1 cup tomato sauce
1 tablespoon chopped fresh flat-leaf parsley
salt and freshly-ground black pepper

1. Pre-heat oven to 400 degrees.
2. Wash the mullet then roll in flour seasoned with salt and pepper.
3. Place the oil in a roasting pan and heat in the oven. Arrange the fish in the hot oil and brown in the oven for about 8 minutes. Remove and turn the fish over. Be careful not to break the fish while turning it.
4. Add parsley, crushed garlic and tomato sauce. Retun to the oven and cook for 10 minutes longer or until the fish is done.
5. Serve hot with some of the sauce on each of the fish.

Serves 6

Meat and Poultry

In most Italian meals, portions of meat are modest because they are mostly served as a second course (secondo). They usually follow a course of pasta and are accompanied by a salad or vegetables. Veal, lamb, pork and poultry are all favorites in Italy. Opt for fresh (not frozen) meats, with very little fat and cook them within 2-3 days from purchase. Let the meats rest at room temperature for about ½ hour before cooking to give them an opportunity to reconstitute their original textures. If you try cooking meat when it is cold you'll end up with a tough and fibrous taste.

Eldo's Saltimbocca Alla Romana

8 medium veal escalops
8 small slices Prosciutto di Parma
8 leaves fresh sage
2 tablespoons butter
1 tablespoon extra-virgin olive oil
1/3 cup fresh or canned chicken stock, warmed
salt and freshly-ground black pepper

1. Pound the veal slices with a mallet into thin slices. Top with a slice of prosciutto and a sage leaf. Season with salt and pepper and shape the escalops into a roll. Secure each roll with a toothpick.
2. Heat half of the oil and half the butter in a medium-sized skillet. When the butter begins to bubble, add the veal rolls in one layer. Cook for about 5 to 10 minutes, being careful to brown them on all sides.
3. Add the remaining butter, oil and the chicken stock to the pan. Bring to a boil and scrape up the brown residue on the bottom of the skillet with a wooden spoon. Pour the sauce over the veal rolls and serve on a warmed plate.

Serves 4 to 8

The name "saltimbocca" suggests that the veal rolls in this recipe are so good that they do not require a fork and will simply "jump into your mouth." The secret to this dish is using very tender and lean veal. Italian cooks opt for "vitello di latte" from Lombardy. It comes from calves that are fed only on milk and are slaughtered at just a few weeks of age. At the butcher's, look for cuts that are slightly rosy and a fine-grained flesh. No traces of fat should be present.

Roast Veal

The best cuts to buy for this roast are leg, loin or boneless shoulder.

3 lb. round roast
2 garlic cloves, cut into small slivers
¼ cup extra-virgin olive oil
2 tablespoons butter
1 bunch flat-leafed parsley
2 sprigs rosemary
salt and freshly-ground black pepper
2 cups dry red wine
1/3 cup chicken stock

1. Pierce the veal with a sharp knife and insert slivers of garlic.
2. Heat the butter and oil in a large casserole and brown the meat on all sides.
3. Chop the rosemary and parsley and add to the casserole along with the salt, pepper and red wine.
4. Cover and cook in the oven at 350 degrees for about 1¼ hours. If necessary, add a little warm water during cooking.
5. When the meat is cooked, transfer it to a board and cut it into thin slices. Arrange it on a warmed plate.
6. Add the chicken stock to the casserole and heat through to loosen the brown residue. Pour over the roast and serve.

Serves 6

Spezzatino
(Chopped casserole meat)

Spezzatino is the Italian word for "beef stew." It can be made in a variety of ways, but here is my family's favorite. On a cold winter's day, serve it with polenta or mashed potatoes.

2 lb. stewing meat, cut into bite-sized cubes
2 tablespoons flour
4 tablespoons olive oil
1 medium onion, chopped
1 lb. stewed tomatoes
1 cup beef stock
1 cup dry red wine
3 garlic cloves, cut into slivers
2 cups frozen peas
1 teaspoon sugar
salt and freshly-ground black pepper
2 sprigs fresh rosemary

1. Put the flour in a shallow dish and season the flour with salt, pepper and rosemary. Coat the beef cubes evenly with the flour.
2. Heat the oil in a large casserole and brown the beef on all sides over medium heat. Remove the meat and drain it on paper towels.
3. Add the onion to the casserole and scrape the base of the pot to loosen any residue from the meat. Cook for 3 to 4 minutes until the onion begins to soften.
4. Stir in the stewed tomatoes, stock, wine and garlic. Bring to a boil. Return the meat to the casserole and cook (covered) in the oven for 1 to 1½ hours at 325 degrees.
5. Add the peas and sugar in the last 10 minutes of cooking. When the meat is tender, taste the seasonings and adjust if necessary.

Serves 6

Roast Lamb

This is a very simple lamb roast that owes much of its wonderful flavor to fresh herbs and garlic. Serve it with lightly cooked fresh vegetables such as spinach or carrots.

4 lb. leg of lamb with all excess fat trimmed off
5 tablespoons extra-virgin olive oil
4 cloves garlic, cut into slivers
2 sprigs fresh sage
2 sprigs fresh thyme
1 cup dry white wine
2 sprigs fresh rosemary
salt and freshly-ground black pepper

1. Using a sharp knife, make small cuts all around the meat and insert slivers of garlic. Rub the meat with olive oil and seasonings
2. Rub the fresh herbs all over the lamb and transfer it to a baking pan.
3. Roast the lamb for about 45 minutes at 375 degrees. Baste occasionally with the wine. When the meat is cooked, place it on a heated serving dish.
4. Skim any fat away from the pan juices and use the juices as a sauce for the lamb.

Serves 6 to 8

Pork with Marsala and Porcini Mushrooms

2 oz. Porcini mushrooms
8 pork escalops
1 tablespoon balsamic vinegar
8 garlic cloves
2 tablespoons butter
6 tablespoons marsala wine
3 springs fresh rosemary
salt and freshly-ground black pepper

1. Reconstitute the dried mushrooms by letting them stand in a bowl with some hot water.
2. Boil the garlic cloves in a small pan of boiling water until soft (about 10 minutes). Drain and put aside.
3. Brush the pork with the vinegar and season with salt and pepper.
4. Melt the butter in a large skillet and quickly brown the pork on both sides.
5. Add the marsala, rosemary, mushrooms, a few tablespoons of the mushroom water and the garlic.
6. Simmer gently for about 5 minutes until the meat is cooked. Adjust the seasoning, if needed, and serve hot.

Serves 8

Marsala wine is widely used in Italy in veal and poultry dishes. It has a sweet and musky flavor and comes from a city in the west of Sicily from which it takes its name. Try substituting it in any American recipes that normally call for sherry. Unlike sherry, Marsala does not deteriorate once the bottle is opened, so it keeps for a long time in your pantry. The second "secret" ingredient in this recipe is Porcini mushrooms. These mushrooms are meaty in texture and have a fine aromatic flavor. They are expensive to buy, but you'll find that a little goes a long way.

Spring Chicken in Red Wine

A light salad such as arugula or watercress will make a perfect accompaniment to this very robust dish.

3 lb. spring chicken, cut into small pieces
¼ cup extra-virgin olive oil
¾ lb. button onions
flour
3 tablespoons butter
3 tablespoons cognac
½ cup red wine
2 bay leaves
1 cup chicken stock
1 tablespoon flat leafed parsley, chopped
salt and freshly-ground black pepper

1. Sauté the button onions in a little oil. Season with salt and pepper.
2. Flour the chicken pieces lightly. Melt 2 tablespoons of the butter in a second pan. Cook the chicken until golden on all sides.
3. Transfer the onions to the pan with the chicken and check the seasonings. Add the cognac. Flame and then add the wine and bay leaves.
4. When the juices come to a boil, add the chicken stock and simmer for about 45 minutes.
5. When the meat is done, transfer it to a heated serving dish.
6. Scrape any residue from the bottom of the pan. Add 2 tablespoons flour and 1 tablespoon butter to make a smooth and creamy sauce.
7. Pour over the chicken. Then sprinkle it with parsley and serve.

Serves 6

Quail with Grapes

8 quails, washed and cleaned
4 tablespoons extra-virgin olive oil
¼ cup pancetta or bacon, cut in cubes
1 cup dry white wine
1 cup chicken stock
salt and freshly-ground black pepper
8 oz. green grapes

1. Season the inside of the quail with salt and pepper.
2. Heat the oil in a large pan and add the pancetta or bacon. Cook for 4 to 5 minutes.
3. Add the quail to the pan and brown them on all sides. Pour in the wine and cook over medium heat. When the juices are reduced to half, turn the quail over and add the stock. Cook for another 20 to 25 minutes until the meat becomes tender.
4. Transfer the quail to a heated plate. Spoon off any fat remaining in the pan and pour the remaining sauce in a small saucepan.
5. Blanch the grapes in a pan of boiling water for a few minutes. Drain and add the grapes to the saucepan. Warm them gently for 3 minutes and spoon around the quail. Serve hot.

Serves 4 to 8

Quail has a very delicate, gamey flavor and benefits from the sweet added flavoring of grapes. These birds are very small so you may want to serve 2 per person or accompany them with a generous serving of vegetables.

DESSERTS

Flavored ice desserts
are a great way to
keep desserts light
and very refreshing.
The following
version is made ·
with coffee, a
personal favorite,
but you can also
make it with lemon,
peaches, orange,
watermelon,
raspberries or mint.

Dessert is fine once in a while but not as part of everyday meals. Italians usually end meals with a piece of fresh fruit or sorbet. Cakes, ice creams and cookies are eaten in small portions and only at dinner parties, on special occasions or after a Sunday meal. Desserts should be light whenever possible and not mistaken for foods that are supposed to provide nourishment.

Granita (Shaved Ice)

1 ½ cups water
½ cup sugar
2 cups espresso coffee

1   Dissolve the sugar into the hot coffee soon after it is made. Allow it to cool completely.
2.   Add the water and stir well. Pour into a shallow container and freeze until solid.
3.   Turn the frozen mixture out onto a board and chop into chunks.
4.   Place the chunks into a food processor and process until smooth. Pour into tall glasses and serve immediately.

Serves 4

Hazelnut Gelato

¾ cup hazelnuts
3 cups milk
3 vanilla beans
6 egg yolks
½ cup sugar

1. Toast the hazelnuts on a cookie sheet under a broiler for 5 to 7 minutes.
2. Allow to cool and then remove their dark skin using a clean dish towel.
3. Grind the nuts in a food processor with 3 tablespoons sugar. The sugar will absorb some of the oils and keep the nuts from turning into a mushy mess.
4. In a saucepan, heat the milk with the vanilla beans. Remove it from the heat just when small bubbles appear on the surface. Do not let the milk boil. Allow the milk to cool.
5. Beat the eggs with a whisk or beater. Add the sugar and continue to beat for a few minutes longer. Gradually add the milk through a strainer in order to discard the vanilla beans.
6. Give the mixture a good stir and then pour in a double boiler. Add the chopped nuts and stir frequently until the custard begins to thicken. Remove from the heat and allow to cool completely in the refridgerator. Freeze in an ice-cream maker according to the manufacturer's directions.

Serves 4 to 6

Gelato is the Italian version of ice cream. However, Italian gelato has much less fat, less cream and less sugar than ice cream made in the United States. Hazelnut-flavored gelato is one of many very popular flavors.

Ricotta Pudding

This pudding is very popular in Sicily. This version is very easy to make and can be made many hours in advance before you are planning to serve it. You can omit the liqueur for a wonderful pudding for children.

1½ cup ricotta cheese
1 cup heavy cream, pasteurized but not ultra-pasteurized
¼ cup sugar
¼ cup sweet Marsala
finely-grated rind of 1 orange or 1 lemon
strips of thinly pared orange or lemon rind to decorate
Optional: ½ cup candied fruits

1. In a bowl, combine the ricotta with the Marsala, sugar and orange or lemon rind.
2. In a separate bowl, whip the cream until soft peaks begin to form.
3. Fold the whipped cream into the ricotta mixture. Spoon into individual bowls and chill until ready to serve. Decorate with the rinds.

Serves 6

Patrizia's Tiramisù

8 oz. light cream cheese
4 oz. mascarpone cheese
1 cup light cream, pasteurized but not ultra-pasteurized
1/3 cup sugar
3 egg yolks
1/3 cup sweet Marsala liqueur
1 cup cooled espresso coffee (use an Italian brand)
3 tablespoons unsweetened Dutch cocoa
24 *savoiardi* cookies

1. In an electric mixer, beat the cream cheese and the mascarpone cheese until soft. Add the cream, sugar, and egg yolks and beat them with the cheese until the mixture turns into soft peaks.
2. In a shallow dish combine the coffee and liquor. Dip each of the *savoiardi* in this mixture just enough to saturate. Be careful not to leave them in too long or they will disintegrate.
3. Line the bottom of an 8-inch glass baking dish with a single layer of coffee-soaked *savoiardi.* Then spread 1/3 of the cheese mixture over the soaked *savoiardi.* Place another layer of *savoiardi* on top of the cheese mixture. Continue with additional alternating layers until you have used all of the *savoiardi* and cheese mixture.
4. Sprinkle with cocoa powder, cover and refrigerate overnight.

Serves 8

The name tiramisú translates into "pick-me-up." This means that if you are feeling down, this dessert will lighten your spirits. Classic tiramisú is made with mascarpone cheese and fresh egg yolks which is, unfortunately, 90% fat. Be careful, therefore, not to indulge in this dessert too often. This version uses a combination of light cream cheese and mascarpone and is lighter in calories.

Italian Pound Cake

This delicious pound cake is perfect served plain or dusted with a bit of confectioner's sugar. You can also replace the orange juice with milk and the orange extract with vanilla or other flavoring for a different tasting cake.

4 eggs, separated
½ lb. unsalted butter, softened
2 cups sugar
1 teaspoon orange extract
2¼ cups flour
a pinch of salt
2 teaspoons baking powder
1 cup orange juice

1. Preheat oven to 350 degrees.
2. Grease and flour a 9 x 3 inch springfoam pan.
3. Beat egg whites with an electric mixer until stiff.
4. In second large bowl, cream the butter with the sugar and orange extract. Add the egg yolks one at a time, beating well after each one.
5. In a third bowl, combine the flour, salt and baking powder. Then add the flour mixture and the orange juice to the bowl with the butter and sugar a little at a time, alternating between the flour and the juice.
6. Carefully fold in the egg whites.
7. Pour batter into the baking pan. Bake for 1 hour or more until done.
8. Allow cake to cool completely before slicing and serving. Dust with confectioner's sugar if you like.

Serves 10 to 12

Strawberry Macedonia

1 lb. fresh, ripe strawberries
1 pint blueberries
5 tablespoons fresh lemon juice
½ cup sugar

1. Cut the strawberries into small pieces and place in a glass bowl.
2. Add the blueberries, sugar and fresh lemon juice. Give the mixture a good stir and refrigerate for a few hours before serving.

Serves 6

Macedonie or fruit salads can be made with just about any mixture of fresh seasonal fruits. Just add fresh lemon juice and sugar for taste. A few tablespoons light liquor such as kirsch or maraschino may also be added.

APPENDIX 1:
Calorie Content Table

This chart may be used to check the approximate calorie content of foods we eat every day.

Food	Portion Size	Calorie Value
CEREALS • RICE • BREADS • NOODLES		
Biscotti, almond (all brands)	1 small (2.5 ounces)	55
Bread	1 slice	80
Bread sticks	1 stick (2 ounces)	140
Bread, wheat	1 slice	65
Cereal, hot	½ cup, cooked (1.4 ounces)	130
Chips, potato	20 chips	158
Chips, tortilla	12 chips	141
Crackers, animal	8	136
Crackers, graham	2 2.5-inch crackers	60
Crackers, saltines, large	2 crackers (1 ounce each)	59
English muffin	1 muffin (2 ounces)	134
French fries	1 child's meal (2.6 ounces)	227
Hamburger bun	1 small bun (1.5 ounces)	123
Muffin	1 small (1 ounce)	80
Noodles, egg	½ cup, cooked	107
Oatmeal	½ cup, cooked	73
Pasta	½ cup, cooked (2.5 ounces)	96
Pizza bread, whole wheat	1/6 of a 12-inch circle (2 ounces)	120
Popcorn cakes	2 – 4 inch (.6 ounce)	60
Popcorn, air popped	3 cups	93
Pretzel, hard plain	2 medium twists	46
Rice cakes	2 – 4 inch	70
Rice, white	½ cup, cooked (2.75 ounces)	103
Roll	1 small (1 ounce)	84
Taco shells, corn	2 - 6 inch (1 ounce)	139

Food	Portion Size	Calorie Value
Tortilla, corn	2 - 6 inch (1.7 ounces)	120
Tortilla, flour	2 - 6 inch (3 ounces)	190
FRUITS		
Apple, unpeeled	1 medium (5.5 ounces)	92
Applesauce, unsweetened	½ cup	53
Apricot, raw	3 medium (1.2 ounces each)	50
Apricots, canned in juice	½ cup (4.3 ounces)	59
Apricots, dried	4 halves	34
Banana (ripe)	1 medium (5 ounces)	94
Blueberries	½ cup (2.5 ounces)	41
Cherries, sour red fresh	½ cup (2.75 ounces)	39
Cherries, sweet fresh	½ cup (2.5 ounces)	52
Dates, dried	3 medium (.3 ounce each)	68
Fig, dried	1	48
Fruit cocktail, canned in juice	1 cup (8 ounces)	108
Fruit salad	6 ounces	70
Fruit, dried	1 ounce	69
Grapefruit	½ large (5.8 ounces)	53
Grapes, black	½ cup (1.6 ounces)	31
Grapes, green or red, seedless	½ cup (2.8 ounces)	57
Kiwi, peeled	1 large (3.2 ounces)	56
Mango	½ medium (5.5 ounces)	102
Melon	1/8 medium	56
Melon balls	7 balls (.5 ounce each)	35
Orange	1 medium (5.3 ounces)	69
Papaya, raw	½ small (5.4 ounces)	59
Peach	1 medium (3.5 ounces)	42
Pear	1 medium (5.8 ounces)	98
Pineapple, diced	1 cup (5.5 ounces)	76
Plums	1 medium (2.3 ounces)	36
Pomegranate	1 medium	121
Prunes	3 prunes (.75 ounce)	60
Raisins	2 tablespoons	84
Raspberries	½ cup (2.15 ounces)	30

Food	Portion Size	Calorie Value
Strawberries	½ cup sliced (2.9 ounces)	25
Watermelon	½ cup diced (2.7 ounces)	25
JUICES		
Apple juice	½ cup (4 fluid ounces)	58
Apricot nectar	½ cup (4 fluid ounces)	269
Grape juice	½ cup (4 fluid ounces)	82
Grapefruit juice	½ cup (4 fluid ounces)	63
Lemon juice	2 tablespoons	15
Orange juice	½ cup (4 fluid ounces)	56
Pineapple juice	½ cup (4 fluid ounces)	59
Tomato juice	½ cup (4 fluid ounces)	26
VEGETABLES		
Artichoke	1 large (7 ounces)	111
Artichoke hearts	1 piece (1.5 ounce)	7
Arugula	½ cup (.35 ounce)	3
Asparagus	4 medium spears (2 ounces)	11
Avocado	½ medium (3.5 ounces)	160
Bamboo shoots	½ cup (2 ounces)	7
Basil	5 leaves	1
Bean sprouts	½ cup (2 ounces)	17
Beet greens	½ cup (2.5 ounces)	19
Bok choy	1 bok choy (3 ounces)	11
Broccoli	3 florets (3.5 ounces)	29
Broccoli rabe	1/5 bunch (3 ounces)	30
Brussel sprouts	4 medium (3 ounces)	30
Cabbage	1 cup chopped (3 ounces)	21
Carrots	2 4-inch sticks (3 ounces)	36
Cauliflower	1 cup (3.5 ounces)	25
Celery	3 5-inch stalks (1.5 ounces)	6
Celery root	1 cup, chopped (3.5 ounces)	14
Chard, fresh raw	1 cup (1.2 ounces)	7
Chives, fresh raw	1 tablespoon, chopped	1
Coleslaw	6 ounces	150

Food	Portion Size	Calorie Value
Collard greens	2 cups	25
Cucumber, peeled	1 cup chopped	16
Dandelion greens, fresh raw	½ cup (1 ounce)	13
Eggplant, fresh raw peeled	1/4 medium (4 ounces)	27
Endive, fresh raw	1 cup, chopped (1.8 ounces)	9
Fennel	1 bulb (8 ounces)	73
Green onions	1 tablespoon chopped	2
Green salad, mixed	8 ounces	46
Hearts of palm	1 cup (9 ounces)	50
Kale	1 cup	34
Kohlrabi	1 cup (4.7 ounces)	36
Leeks	¼ cup chopped (.9 ounce)	8
Lettuce	1 cup shredded (1.9 ounces)	8
Lettuce, Romaine	1 cup shredded (1 ounce)	5
Mushrooms, raw	7 medium (.6 ounce each)	28
Okra, boiled, drained	8 3-inch pods	19
Olives, black	10	40
Onion	1 large (8 ounces)	95
Parsley	1 tablespoon, chopped	1
Peas, boiled and drained	¼ cup (1.5 ounces)	36
Pepper, green or red	1 medium (5 ounces)	28
Potato salad	½ cup (4.5 ounces)	199
Potato, baked	1 medium (6 ounces)	161
Potatoes, sweet	1 medium (4 ounces)	103
Pumpkin	½ cup, mashed	42
Radicchio	1 cup, shredded (1.5 ounces)	10
Radishes	2 radishes (3 ounces each)	28
Rhubarb	1 cup, diced (4.3 ounces)	26
Sauerkraut	1 cup (7 ounces)	50
Scallions	½ cup (2 ounces)	18
Snow Peas	9 pods (1 ounce)	10
Spinach	1 bunch (12 ounces)	78
Squash, spaghetti	½ cup (2.75 ounces)	21
Squash, summer	½ cup (2.25 ounces)	12
Tomato	1 medium (5 ounces)	26

Food	Portion Size	Calorie Value
Tomatoes, cherry	5 (.6 ounces each)	25
Turnips	1 cup chopped (5 ounces)	30
Water chestnuts	4 nuts (1.2 ounces)	35
Yams	1 medium 6" (8 ounces)	263
Zucchini	6 slices (4 ounces)	113
Spaghetti sauce	½ cup (4.4 ounces)	72
Vegetable juice	½ cup (4 fluid ounces)	46
Vegetable soup	1 cup (8 fluid ounces)	122
BEANS AND NUTS		
Almonds, dry roasted	24-28 medium whole (1 ounce)	170
Bean soup	1 can (11 oz)	282
Beans, pinto, cooked	½ cup (3 ounces)	122
Cashews, dry roasted	1 ounce	163
Lentils, boiled	1/2 cup (3.5 ounces)	115
Peanut Butter	2 tablespoons	190
Peanuts, roasted	30 large - 60 small (1 ounce)	166
Pistachios	¼ cup, 45 nuts (1 ounce)	158
Walnuts, black	15-20 halves (1 ounce)	176
MILK & MILK PRODUCTS		
Butter	1 tablespoon (.5 ounce)	100
Buttermilk	1 cup (8 fluid ounces)	134
Cheese, cottage, creamed	½ cup (4 ounces)	120
Cheese, mozzarella	1 slice (1 ounce)	72
Cheese, natural	1 ounce	120
Cheese, Parmigiano Reggiano	1 tablespoon	20
Cheese, ricotta, whole milk	¼ cup (2 ounces)	92
Cream cheese	1 tablespoon (.5 ounce)	52
Cream cheese, light	1 tablespoon (.5 ounce)	35
Cream, light (30% fat)	2 tablespoons (1 fluid ounce)	88
Cream, heavy (37% fat)	2 tablespoons, 1/4 cup whipped, (1 fluid ounce)	104
Cream, sour	2 tablespoons (1 fluid ounce)	64

Food	Portion Size	Calorie Value
Cream, sour, light	2 tablespoons (1 fluid ounce)	41
Ice cream, vanilla	½ cup	140
Milk, whole	1 cup (8 fluid ounces)	144
Milk, 2% fat	1 cup (8 fluid ounces)	122
Milk, non-fat	1 cup (8 fluid ounces)	88
Milk, dried, reconstituted	1 cup (8 fluid ounces)	80
Milk, evaporated	½ cup (4 fluid ounces)	161
Milkshake	small (12 fluid ounces)	540
Soy Milk	1 cup (8 fluid ounces)	105
Yogurt, plain, fat-free	1 cup (8 ounces)	138
Yogurt, frozen, fat-free	1/2 cup (3 ounces)	91
SUGAR • SWEETS • SPREADS		
Artificial Sweetener	1 gram packet	0
Honey	2 tablespoons	128
Ice cream, vanilla	1/2 cup	140
Jam/ marmalade	1 tablespoon	49
Milk chocolates	1 bar (.6 ounce)	91
Sugar	1 tablespoon	48
CAKES/ PASTRIES		
Angel food cake	1 slice (2 ounces)	120
Apple pie	1/8 of a 9-inch pie (4.5 ounces)	340
Brownie	1 piece (3.5 ounces)	430
Cake, white, without frosting	1/12 cake (1.5 ounces)	238
Cake, chocolate, without frosting	1/12 cake (1.5 ounces)	273
Chocolate chip cookie	1 large (2.5 ounces)	275
Custard made with 2% milk	1/2 cup (4.7 ounces)	149
Frosting	2 tablespoons	130
Fruit cake	1/28 cake (1.5 ounces)	336
Pumpkin pie	1/8 of a 9-inch pie (4 ounces)	240

Food	Portion Size	Calorie Value
OILS		
Mayonnaise	1 tablespoon	100
Olive	1 tablespoon	124
Vegetable / Corn	1 tablespoon	126
WHITE MEAT		
Drained, canned fish	2 to 3 ounces	99
Turkey frankfurter	1 (1.5 ounces)	80
Turkey ham	1 ounce	36
Cooked poultry, without skin or bones, broiled/grilled	1 small breast (4.9 ounces)	231
FISH		
Cooked fish, without bones	3 ounces	128
Mussels	3.5 ounces	170
Octopus, cooked	3 ounces	141
Oysters, raw	6 medium	240
Shrimp, cooked	6 large	33
Squid, fried	3.5 ounces	175
RED MEAT		
Cooked lean beef, pork, or lamb without bones	3 ounces	232
Beef or pork frankfurter	1 (1.6 ounce)	140
Lean ham, roasted	3 ounce	141
Pancetta	1 ounce	100
Prosciutto	1 ounce	70
EGGS		
1 egg, extra large	1 yolk and one egg white (1.76 ounces)	75
1 egg white	1 large egg white	17

Food	Portion Size	Calorie Value
BEVERAGES		
80 proof alcohol	1 fluid ounce	69
Beer	12 fluid ounces	148
Clear broth/bouillon	1 cup (8 fluid ounces)	38
Club soda	1 1/2 cups (12 fluid ounces)	1
Coffee, regular or decaffeinated	1 cup prepared (8 fluid ounces)	5
Diet soda	12 fluid ounces	2
Herb tea (without barley or any fruit sugar added)	1 bag, prepared (.7 ounce)	0
Sparkling water	12 fluid ounces	0
Tea	1 cup prepared (8 fluid ounces)	1
Wine	5 fluid ounces	106
MISC		
Chewing gum (sugarless)	1 stick	10

Source: calorieking.com

APPENDIX 2:
Exercise Flow Chart

PERSONAL INFORMATION

Name: _____Age: _____

☐   Male   ☐   Female

Emergency contact:_____   Phone: _____

Doctor's name: _____   Phone: _____

PHYSICAL ACTIVITY: ARE YOU READY?	Yes	No
1. Has a doctor ever said you have heart trouble?	☐	☐
2. Do you frequently suffer from pains in your chest?	☐	☐
3. Do you often feel faint or have spells of severe dizziness?	☐	☐
4. Do you have high blood pressure?	☐	☐
5. Has a doctor ever told you that you have a bone or joint problem, such as arthritis or bursitis, back or knee problems, that can be made worse by exercise?	☐	☐
6. Do you have uncontrolled asthma?	☐	☐
7. Do you have diabetes?	☐	☐
8. Do you have high cholesterol?	☐	☐
9. Have you had recent surgery?	☐	☐
10. Do you get short of breath easily?	☐	☐
11. Do you have a hernia?	☐	☐
12. Are you over age 65?	☐	☐
13. Have you consulted your doctor about an exercise program?	☐	☐
14. Will you consult your physician before increasing your physical activity and/or take a fitness evaluation?	☐	☐

Please list any medications/supplements you are currently taking

Name of Medication	Dosage	Reason for Taking
_____	_____	_____
_____	_____	_____
_____	_____	_____
_____	_____	_____
_____	_____	_____

☐   I do not take prescription or over-the-counter medication.

Structural Assessment
Postural Analysis
Standing alignment is effective when the weight bearing joints fall within the body's line of gravity.

Head	Shoulder Girdle	Pelvis	Knees	Feet
☐ Level	☐ Joint centered	☐ Level	☐ Straight in	☐ Pointing forward
☐ Centered	☐ Scapula movement	☐ Normal lordotic curve	☐ Patella centered	☐ Normal arch
	☐ Shoulders level			
	☐ Elbows pointing back			

Goal Assessment

Date						
	Start	Goal	30 day	60 day	90 day	120 day
Height						
Weight						
Blood pressure						
Resting pulse						
Max H.R.						
Mean H.R.						
Step/cardio test						
Sit & reach test						
Trunk strength						
Push up (60 sec)						

Body Composition

Date						
	Start	Goal	30 day	60 day	90 day	120 day
Thigh (MF)						
Pec (M) Triceps (F)						
Abs (M) Hip (F)						
Bicep						
Tricep						
Body fat %						
Lbs. fat mass						
Lbs. lean mass						

Circumference Measurements

Date						
	Start	Goal	30 day	60 day	90 day	120 day
Chest						
Upper arm						
Waist						
Hip						
Thigh						
Calf						

1. Caloric Goal_____

2. Need diet or nutrition? _____

3. Aerobic exercise   Time_____   Jogging

                         _____   Eliptical

                         _____   Bicycle

4. Anaerobic exercise   Time_____   Chest

                         _____   Abdomen

                         _____   Arm

                         _____   Legs

                         _____   Back

APPENDIX 3:
Post Bariatric Surgery Diet

This is a four-phase diet that has been developed to help my patients who have had bariatric surgery, such as gastric bypass, sleeve gastrectomy, gastroplasty, or gastric banding. Because the size of their stomach has been reduced, they need to learn how to eat all over again, starting with a very light intake of foods and graduating to larger portions with more complex foods. You may follow this diet if you wish to lose a large amount of weight fairly quickly. The end goal of weight loss surgery is to lose approximately 70% of total body fat. However, you will not need to lose this extreme an amount of weight. You can follow some of the principles used by my surgery patients to lose weight, but please remember that this is not a permanent diet and no substitute for permanently changing your eating patterns. After you have lost a large amount of weight, you should follow the healthy eating plan outlined in the modified Italian diet presented in this book.

Diet Principles:

Because of the reduced stomach size after bariatric surgery, the amount of food allowed at any given time is limited to no more than 1 – 2 ounces every 30-60 minutes. High caloric foods, beverages, or snacks are omitted from this plan. It is recommended that food be eaten slowly and in very small quantities at meal times. You should allow at least 20-30 minutes for each meal. You are encouraged to drink 6 cups of fluid a day to prevent dehydration. You should sip one cup of water over the period of one hour. Stop sipping liquids at least 45-60 minutes before meals. Because the caloric intake is low and food choices are limited, it is difficult to meet your body's need for vitamins and minerals; therefore, you should take a multivitamin/mineral supplement that provides 100% of the RDA in the form of a chewable tablet or liquid supplement. Foods need to be chewed very well to prevent obstruction. Food should be chewed to the consistency of applesauce.

You may follow this diet if you wish to lose a large amount of weight fairly quickly, but this is not a permanent diet and no substitute for permanently changing your eating habits.

Phase I Food Plan
First Two Weeks Post Surgery
Full Liquids

Phase I Food Plan Examples

Water
Iced tea
Popsicles
Frozen Fruit Pops
Clear broth (Watch for high salt content.)
Sports drinks
Crystal light
Unsweetened juices

Suggestions

1. Freeze plastic bottles with desired liquids ahead of time to carry with you.
2. Continue with 60 cc of liquid every 30 minutes but increase as you are able to tolerate more liquids. The goal is to drink six 8-ounce glasses a day.
3. Using a spoon may help. Be careful to measure all liquids.
4. Do not gulp liquids or drink quickly. This can cause stomach pain and intense nausea.

Phase II Food Plan

2-6 Weeks Post Surgery
Soft Foods

Phase II Food Plan Examples

Oatmeal, cream of wheat, or Malt-o Meal with skim milk*
Thinned mashed potatoes
Pureed foods
Baked potato
Canned fruit (no pineapple at this time)
Poached or soft boiled egg*
Applesauce
Cottage cheese*
Yogurt
Low-fat cream soups
Protein powder. (If lactose intolerant, try 1-2 scoops of SOYA* in juice.)
One packet Carnation Instant Breakfast, if desired*

During this phase, you will only need to eat one meal, twice a day. In the beginning, you may only be able to tolerate 1-2 tablespoons at a time. You must chew foods slowly and completely. Eat in a relaxed setting; eat slowly and without interruptions. Use a small saucer or a child-size cup to measure food. Fill the cup to ½ full with food. Do not drink liquids 30 minutes before meals or 1 hour after meals.

* Denotes food high in protein.

In this phase, it is not only important to continue with your fluid intake, but also to incorporate protein-rich foods into your diet. You want to obtain 60–90 grams of protein a day.

Phase III Food Plan

6 weeks to 6 months
Semi-Soft Foods
200-300 calorie
60 grams protein

Phase III Food Plan Examples

Tuna fish *
Whitefish *
Shrimp, lobster, crab *
Lean ground beef *
Chicken *
Peanut butter *
Pasta
Canned soups (low salt)
Vegetables/Salads
Fresh fruits
Crackers, graham crackers
Poached or boiled eggs *
Protein bars *

Cook all foods without adding fats. Broil, bake, or poach meats, fish, and poultry. Season vegetables with herbs and spices; do not use butter, margarine, or other fats. Some spices may cause stomach upset. You may need to introduce these slowly to your diet. These include red, green or black peppers, chili powder, vinegars, and other spices.

** Remember to stop eating when you feel full.
* Denotes foods that are good sources of protein.

Phase IV Food Plan
Solids
200-300 calories
60 to 90 grams of protein

Phase IV Food Plan Examples

Chicken, ½ to full breast (baked or broiled)
4-5 scoops cottage or ricotta cheese *
2 oz. lean ground beef or soft cooked beef *
3 oz. tuna or fish *
Shrimp, lobster, crab (less than 2 ounces*)
Peanut butter, 3 ounces
All vegetables, ½ cup
All fruits, ½ cup
3 oz. of eggs, cooked without fat *
All cereals, ½ cup
Salad, ½ - ¼ cup
Potatoes, ½ to 1 whole baked, ½ cup mashed
Pasta, ¼ to ½ cup
Crackers, graham crackers
Protein bars
Protein powder or SOYA powder

Prepare foods as described in the Phase III Food Plan.

*Denotes foods that are good sources of protein.

APPENDIX 4:
Important Tips when Dieting

- There is no painless way to melt away pounds. Your total calories eaten must be less than the total calories expended in order for you to lose weight.
- Avoid overeating. Stop when you are full.
- Chew foods thoroughly. 30 chews per bite.
- Use small bowls, plates, and spoons.
- Put your fork or spoon down in between bites.
- Drink 8-10 cups of liquids per day, in between meals.
- Do not drink high-calorie drinks such as milkshakes, cokes, beer, or other alcoholic beverages.
- Do not forget to take vitamins 3-4 times per day.
- Do not eat high-calorie, low-nutrient foods such as cake, cookies, candy, pastries, jam, jellies, honey, sugar, or ice cream.
- Bake, broil, or steam foods instead of frying them to cut down on empty calories.
- Exercise!
- Do not watch TV or talk while eating your meal as this will distract you and make you less aware of your body signaling that you are full.

APPENDIX 5:
High-Protein Foods

Below is a list of some common foods and their protein content.

Serving Size	Protein (grams)
Almonds (1 cup)	26.0
Hamburger (3 oz.)	21.8
Roast beef (3 oz.)	23.3
Beef pot pie	23.0
Cottage cheese (½ cup)	13.6
Chicken (½ breast)	24.7
Chicken drumstick	12.5
Chicken, dark (3.5 oz.)	29.3
Chicken, white (3.5 oz.)	32.3
Chicken pot pie	23.0
Chicken salad (½ cup)	17.4
Cocoa from mix	7.4
Corn bread (1 square)	5.0
Cream soups (1 cup)	7.0
Custard (½ cup)	7.2
Egg, boiled	6.3
Egg	6.7
Egg, scrambled	7.1
Baked flounder	30.2
Haddock (1 fillet)	16.6
Red snapper (3 oz.)	39.0
Scallops (5-6 med.)	39.5
Shrimp (5 large)	15.5
Baked ham (3 oz.)	26.3
Boiled ham (2 oz.)	14.5
Lamb chop (4 oz.)	20.2
Lobster (1 cup)	19.5
Skim milk (1 cup)	8.0
Peanut butter (1 tablespoon.)	8.5
Pork chops (3.5 oz.)	21.4
Broiled trout (3 oz.)	20.3
Water-packed tuna (½ cup)	36.4
Turkey, dark (3.5 oz.)	30.0
Turkey, white (3.5 oz.)	32.9
Chocolate pudding (1 cup)	8.1
Yogurt (½ cup)	4.4

References

Hu FB, Stampfer MJ, Manson JE, Rimm EB, Colditz GA, Rosner BA, Speizer FE, Hennekens CH, Willett WC. Frequent Nut Consumption and Risk of Coronary Heart Disease in Women: Prospective Cohort Study. British Medical Journal 1998 November 14; 317 (7169): 1341-5.

Keys A, Taylor HL, Blackburn H, Brozek J, Anderson JT, Simonson E. Coronary Heart Disease Among Minnesota Business and Professional Men Followed 15 Years. Circulation 1963; 28: 381-95.

NIH Consensus: Gastrointestinal surgery for severe obesity. National Institute of Health Consensus Development Conference Draft Statement. Obes Surg. 1991;1:257-65.

Olshansky SJ, Passaro DJ, Hershow RC, Layden J, Carnes BA, Brody J, Hayflick L, Butler RN, Allison DB, Ludwig DS. A Potential Decline in Life Expectancy in the United States in the 21st Century. New England Journal of Medicine 2005 March 17; 352: 1138-1145.

Tudor-Locke C, Pangrazi RP, Corbin CB, Rutherford WJ, Vincent SD, Raustorp A, Tomson LM, Cuddihy TF. BMI-Referenced Standards for Recommended Pedometer-Determined Steps/Day in Children. Preventive Medicine 2004 June; 38 (6); 857-64.

World Health Organization. Health Systems: Improving Performance. The World Health Report 2000. Geneva: WHO, 2000.

Frezza EE. Are We Closer to Finding the Treatment for Type II Diabetes Mellitus in Morbid Obesity? Are Incretins the Key to Success? Obesity Surgery 2004; 14:999-1005.

Frezza, EE. New Concepts of Physiology in Obese Patients. Digestive Diseases and Sciences. 2004 June; 49(6):1062-1064

Frezza EE, et al. Laparoscopic re-exploration in mechanical bowel obstruction after laparoscopic gastric bypass for morbid obesity. Minerva Chirurgica. 2006;61(3):193-7.

Frezza EE, et al. Laparoscopic Gastric Bypass for Morbid Obesity Decreases Bodily Pain, Improves Physical Functioning and Mental Health in Women. JLAST. In press.

Frezza EE, et al. Morbid Obesity Causes Increased Intraabdominal Pressure. Digestive Diseases and Sciences. In press.

Frezza EE, et al. The Multiple Faces of Glucagon-Like Peptide 1-Obesity, Appetite, and Stress: What Is Next? A Review. Digestive Diseases and Sciences. In press.

Frezza EE. Laparoscopic Vertical Sleeve Gastrectomy For Morbid Obesity. Where Are We Going? A Review. Surgery Today. In Press.

The Author

Dr. Eldo E. Frezza was born and raised in Italy. He is currently professor and the Director of the Bariatric Weight Loss Center and Chief of General Surgery at Texas Tech University Health Science Center.

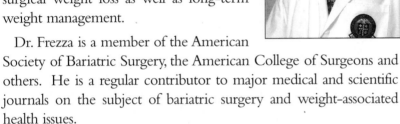

In his practice he has treated thousands of patients for both their surgical and non-surgical weight loss as well as long-term weight management.

Dr. Frezza is a member of the American Society of Bariatric Surgery, the American College of Surgeons and others. He is a regular contributor to major medical and scientific journals on the subject of bariatric surgery and weight-associated health issues.

He lives in Texas with his wife and two sons.